Hochschulschriften

Institut für Systembiotechnologie
Universität des Saarlandes

Herausgegeben von Prof. Dr. Christoph Wittmann

Band 7

I0131848

Cuvillier-Verlag
Göttingen, Deutschland

Herausgeber
Univ.-Prof. Dr. Christoph Wittmann
Institut für Systembiotechnologie
Universität des Saarlandes
Campus A1.5, 66123 Saarbrücken
www.iSBio.de

Hinweis: Obgleich alle Anstrengungen unternommen wurden, um richtige und aktuelle Angaben in diesem Werk zum Ausdruck zu bringen, übernehmen weder der Herausgeber, noch der Autor oder andere an der Arbeit beteiligten Personen eine Verantwortung für fehlerhafte Angaben oder deren Folgen. Eventuelle Berichtigungen können erst in der nächsten Auflage berücksichtigt werden.

Bibliographische Informationen der Deutschen Nationalbibliothek
Die Deutsche Nationalbibliothek verzeichnet diese Publikation in der Deutschen Nationalbibliographie; detaillierte bibliographische Daten sind im Internet über *http://dnb.d-nb.de* abrufbar.
1. Aufl. – Göttingen: Cuvillier, 2018

© Cuvillier-Verlag · Göttingen 2018
   Nonnenstieg 8, 37075 Göttingen
   Telefon: 0551-54724-0
   Telefax: 0551-54724-21
   www.cuvillier.de

1. Auflage, 2018
Gedruckt auf umweltfreundlichem, säurefreiem Papier aus nachhaltiger Forstwirtschaft.

ISBN 978-3-7369-9913-8
eISBN 978-3-7369-8913-9
ISSN 2199-7756

Metabolic engineering of *Basfia succiniciproducens* for the production of carbon-three compounds

Dissertation

zur Erlangung des Grades

des Doktors der Naturwissenschaften

der Naturwissenschaftlich-Technischen Fakultät

der Universität des Saarlandes

von

Jonathan Thomas Fabarius

Saarbrücken

2018

Tag des Kolloquiums: 9. November 2018

Dekan: Prof. Dr. Guido Kickelbick

Berichterstatter: Prof. Dr. Christoph Wittmann

Prof. Dr. Elmar Heinzle

Vorsitz: Prof. Dr. Gert-Wieland Kohring

Akad. Mitarbeiter: Dr. Björn Becker

PUBLICATIONS

Partial results of this work have been published previously. This was authorized by the Institute of Systems Biotechnology, represented by Prof. Dr. Christoph Wittmann.

Peer-reviewed articles

Becker J., Lange A., **Fabarius J.**, Wittmann C., (2015). Top value platform chemicals: bio-based production of organic acids. Current Opinion in Biotechnology 36: 168-175.

Patents

Krawczyk, J. M., Haefner, S., Schröder, H., Zelder, O., **Fabarius, J. T.** (2015). Modified microorganism for improved production of alanine. Application No./Patent No. PCT/IB2014/063950

CONTRIBUTION

Students

Parts of this published work were contributed by the following students under supervision.

Nadja Barton constructed in her master's thesis "Molekularbiologische Studien mit *Basfia succiniciproducens* zur Optimierung der Stammentwicklung" the strain *B. succiniciproducens* DD3ΔDD0759ΔDD0810, by deletion of the *DD0810* and *DD0759 lacZ* genes. Furthermore, complementation of the latter gene function was proven with the constructed plasmids Bsuc_PL18 and Bsuc_PL19. These plasmids contain the *lacZ* genes *DD0810* and *DD0759* under native promoter control, respectively. Additionally, the construction of the promoter screening plasmids Bsuc_PL8, Bsuc_PL9, Bsuc_PL10 and Bsuc_PL11 was conducted in this work.

DANKSAGUNG

Vielen Menschen gilt mein Dank, die mich beim Entstehen dieser Arbeit unterstützt, begleitet und motiviert haben.

Besonders bedanken möchte ich mich bei meinem Doktorvater Professor Dr. Christoph Wittmann für die immer gute Betreuung und die zahlreichen wissenschaftlichen Diskussionen. Deine Ratschläge, Hinweise und dein offenes Ohr haben die Entwicklung meiner Arbeit vereinfacht und das ein oder andere Wort aus meinem Wortschatz getilgt. Danke dafür!

Ebenso möchte ich mich bei den Professoren Elmar Heinzle und Gert-Wieland Kohring für die Übernahme des Zweitgutachtens, beziehungsweise des Prüfungsvorsitzes bedanken.

Auch gilt mein Dank den Mitgliedern der Kooperationsgemeinschaft mit der BASF SE. Hier danke ich Dr. Marvin Schulz, Dr. Stefan Haefner, Dr. Hartwig Schröder, Dr. Joanna-Martyna Krawczyk, Dr. Birgit Hoff und Prof. Dr. Oskar Zelder für den Austausch über die Eigenheiten von *Basfia succiniciproducens*, die gute Kooperation und die finanzielle Unterstützung dieser Arbeit.

Ganz besonderer Dank gilt Dr. Judith Becker und Dr. Michael Kohlstedt, die mir mit Rat, Tat und Humor zur Seite standen. Insbesondere die eine oder andere nächtliche Fermentation wird noch lange im Gedächtnis bleiben. Cola ist gesund.

Auch bei den Mitarbeitern des Instituts für Systembiotechnologie der Universität des Saarlandes bedanke ich mich für die angenehme Zeit und die experimentelle, moralische und freundschaftliche Unterstützung. Ganz besonders danke ich René Bücker, Lisa Dersch, Susanne Schwechheimer, Jessica Stolzenberger und Luise Bücker. Ihr wart maßgeblich verantwortlich für den ein oder anderen legendären Mittwoch-Abend oder auch gelungene Laborspäße. Ein besonderer Dank gebührt auch Gideon Gießelmann (weiterhin durchziehen im Uni-Fit, Gideon!), Rudolf Schäfer, André Luis Rodriguez, Georg Richter und Sarah Schiefelbein für diverse sonnige Stunden auf der Brücke. Unserem HPLC-Spezialisten Michel Fritz danke ich sehr für die stets geduldige Hilfsbereitschaft in HPLC oder GC-MS fragen. Ja. Jetzt war es doch die letzte Messung.

Auch unserer Molekularbiologie-Spezialistin Mirjam Selzer möchte ich danken für Unterstützung, offene Ohren und Ratschläge.

Ein außerordentliches Dankeschön gilt auch meinen Studenten Nadja Barton, Sebastian Baran und Alexander Hammel, die mit ihren Experimenten im Rahmen ihrer Abschlussarbeiten die bearbeitete Thematik bereichert haben, blaues in weißes verwandelten und *Basfia succiniciproducens* zum Leuchten brachten.

Meine zahlreichen Freunde aus Stuttgart, Reutlingen und Saarbrücken die mich motiviert und auch mal auf andere Gedanken gebracht haben, möchte ich nicht unerwähnt lassen. Vielen Dank für gelungene Abende, Diskussionen, Besuche und Streifzüge durch Saarbrücken, Heidelberg, München, Stuttgart und Reutlingen. Ich bin froh, dass es jeden einzelnen von euch gibt.

Auch dir möchte ich danken Laura, dich habe ich hier kennengelernt und möchte dich nicht mehr missen. Danke, dass du mir immer zuhörst und mich aufgemuntert hast, auch mal in eine andere Richtung zu denken. Ich freue mich auf die Zukunft mit dir.

Meinen Eltern danke ich von Herzen für die jahrelange Unterstützung, die Ratschläge und dass sie immer die richtigen Worte parat hatten. Auch meinen beiden Brüdern danke ich für stets motivierende Worte und ihre Hilfe. Ohne euch wäre das Leben nur halb so schön.

Schließen möchte ich mit einem Zitat, das mich schon sehr lange inspiriert:

„Mit Sicherheit werden die Chemiker eines Tages Wege finden, die DNA zu verändern. Wie bei den Kunststoffen wird es eine DNA-Industrie geben. Man wird perfekte DNA herstellen, und die natürliche DNA fälschen, indem man fremde Moleküle einsetzt.
Das eröffnet dem Menschen viele Perspektiven und Hoffnungen.
Aber es entstehen auch Ängste. Ich bin nicht nur Biologe, sondern auch ein Mensch.
Und ich bezweifle, dass der Mensch reif genug ist, die chemische Steuerung seines Schicksals zu übernehmen.

Aber wird er es jemals sein?"

Jean Rostand, 1962

IV

TABLE OF CONTENTS

SUMMARY

The recent rise of bio-succinic acid as industrial platform chemical has brought the rumen bacterium *Basfia succiniciproducens*, a natural producer of this organic acid, into the focus of research. In order to upgrade this industrial producer into a cell factory of broader use, the potential of *B. succiniproducens* to produce carbon-three compounds was explored. A new genome engineering approach and the identification of suitable promoters for gene expression was targeted. For production of the C_3 chemical alanine from glucose and xylose, a bioprocess was developed. Genetic engineering for β-alanine and 3-hydroxypropionate (3-HP) production was examined.

A blue-white selection screening system for genome engineering was established, using a *lacZ* deficient strain. Suitable promoters for heterologous expression of different genes of interest were identified. Using *B. succiniciproducens* ALA-1, hosting a genomic copy of an alanine dehydrogenase from *Geobacillus stearothermophilus*, alanine production was improved to 29 g L^{-1} by establishing a fed-batch strategy under anaerobic conditions. Via equipment of *B. succiniciproducens* with an episomal copy of an aspartate 1-decarboxylase from *Corynebacterium glutamicum* or *Vibrio natriegens*, β-alanine synthesis was realized (450 mg L^{-1}). The expression of a β-alanine pyruvate transaminase from *Pseudomonas putida* and a malonate semialdehyde reductase from *Escherichia coli* enabled production of 3-HP (100 mg L^{-1}) from glucose.

ZUSAMMENFASSUNG

Die Nutzung von Bio-Bernsteinsäure als industrielle Plattformchemikalie hat das Pansen-Bakterium *Basfia succiniciproducens*, einen natürlichen Produzenten dieser organischen Säure, in den Fokus der Forschung gebracht. Um diesen Produzentenstamm für weitere Anwendungen auszubauen, wurde das Potential von *B. succiniciproducens* zur Produktion von C_3 Chemikalien erforscht. Eine neue genombasierte Methode zur genetischen Modifikation sowie geeignete Promotoren für die Genexpression wurden angestrebt. Für die Produktion der C_3 Chemikalie Alanin aus Glucose und Xylose wurde ein Bioprozess entwickelt. Genetische Arbeiten zur Produktion von β-Alanin und 3-Hydroxypropionat (3-HP) wurden durchgeführt.

Ein blau-weiß Screening System für genomische Modifikationen wurde zunächst in einem *lacZ* defizienten Stamm etabliert. Auch geeignete Promotoren für die heterologe Expression verschiedenster Ziel-Gene wurden identifiziert. Der Stamm *B. succiniciproducens* ALA-1, der eine genomische Kopie einer Alanin Dehydrogenase aus *Geobacillus stearothermophilus* besitzt, produzierte 29 g L^{-1} Alanin in einem anaeroben Fed-Batch Prozess. Durch Einbringen von episomalen Kopien einer Aspartat 1-Decarboxylase aus *Corynebacterium glutamicum* oder *Vibrio natriegens* wurde die β-Alanin (450 mg L^{-1}) Synthese realisiert. Die Expression einer β-Alanin Pyruvat Transaminase aus *Pseudomonas putida* und einer Malonate semialdehyd Reduktase aus *Escherichia coli* ermöglichte die Produktion von 3-HP (100 mg L^{-1}) aus Glucose.

1 INTRODUCTION AND OBJECTIVES

1.1 Introduction

Our industrialized world is driven by using fossil resources like petroleum. Mankind's elevated and thriving demand of these non-renewable resources depletes their availability and can lead to shortages with incalculable consequences for our communities and life. Furthermore, the use of fossil resources in our daily life yields a carbon dioxide fingerprint in every single production process of commercial goods or means of transportation (Becker and Wittmann, 2015). This led to elevated carbon dioxide concentrations in our atmosphere (Crutzen, 2002; Dlugokencky and Tans, 2017). Carbon dioxide, as a greenhouse gas, can influence our climate significantly, leading to deviations from its natural behavior (Crutzen, 2002; UNEP, 2017).

To face these challenges and reduce the dependence on fossil resources as well as greenhouse gas emissions, the recent years have seen a tremendous increase in the sustainable production of chemicals and commercial goods through biotechnology processes (Becker et al., 2015; Werpy et al., 2004). Particularly, the production of amino acids (Becker and Wittmann, 2012b) and organic acids (Becker et al., 2015) plays a key role in the development of a bio-based community.

To broaden this further, the US Department of Energy published a candidate list of 12 top value chemicals, which can be derived through biotechnology processes (Werpy et al., 2004). This list comprises carbon-three to carbon-six chemicals, which are grouped into organic acids, amino acids, (sugar) alcohols and lactones. Organic acids are depicted as the bulk fraction of these platform chemicals (**Table 1.1**).

In detail, 3-hydroxypropionate (C_3), the 1,4-diacids succinate, fumarate, malate (C_4), itaconate, levulinate (C_5), 2,5-furandicarboxylate and glucarate (C_6) are mentioned. In particular, amino acids like aspartate (C_4) and glutamate (C_5) are also identified for application in chemical industry. Furthermore, (sugar) alcohols, like the commonly known glycerol (C_3), a side product of biodiesel industry (Yang et al., 2012), and xylitol (xylose, C_5), arabitol (arabinose, C_5) and sorbitol (sorbit, C_6) are listed (Werpy et al., 2004).

Table 1.1. List of top value chemicals comprising compound details and potential applications. Applications are divided in nine categories e.g. industrial. All categories name specific applications e.g. transportation (fuels, anti-freeze, ...). Detailed information is listed in Werpy et al., 2004.

Compound	Compound class	Number of carbon atoms	Derivatives of interest	Application
3-Hydroxypropionate	Organic acid	3	Acrylates, Acrylamides, Esters, 1,3-Propanediol, Malonate	Safe Food Supply, Industrial, Environment, Housing
Glycerol	Sugar alcohol	3	Propylene glycol, Malonate, 1,3-Propanediol, Diacids, Propylalcohol, Dialdehyde, Epoxides	Housing, Industrial, Transportation, Safe Food Supply
Succinate	Organic acid	4	Tetrahydrofuran, 1,4-Butanediol, γ-Butyrolactone, Pyrrolidones, Esters, Diamines, 4,4-Bionelle, Hydroxybutyricacid	Industrial, Textiles, Environment, Transportation, Safe Food Supply, Communication
Aspartate	Amino acid	4	Amino succinate derivatives, Polypyrrolidones	Industrial, Environment, Health and Hygiene
Fumarate	Organic acid	4	Unsaturated succinate derivatives	Transportation, Safe Food Supply, Communication, Housing
Malate	Organic acid	4	Hydroxysuccinate derivatives, Hydroxybutyrolactone	Industrial, Textiles, Environment
Itaconate	Organic acid	5	Methyl succinate derivatives, Unsaturated esters	Transportation, Housing, Textiles, Recreation
Levulinate	Organic acid	5	δ-Aminolevulinate, 2-Methyl Tetrahydrofuran, 1,4-Diols, Esters, Succinate	Industrial, Environment, Health and Hygiene, Textiles, Recreation, Housing
Glutamate	Amino acid	5	Amino diols, Glutarate, Pyrrolidones	Industrial, Textiles, Environment, Safe Food Supply, Health and Hygiene
Xylitol	Sugar alcohol	5	Ethylene glycol, Propylene glycol, Glycerol, Lactate, Hydroxyfurans, Sugar acids	Industrial, Transportation, Safe Food Supply
Arabitol	Sugar alcohol	5		
2,5-Furandicarboxylate	Organic acid	6	Succinate, 2,5-Furan derivatives containing hydroxyl or amino groups	Safe Food Supply, Industrial, Textiles
Glucarate	Organic acid	6	Dilactones, Monolactones, Other products	Industrial, Environment, Health and Hygiene, Housing, Recreation
Sorbitol	Sugar alcohol	6	Ethylene glycol, Propylene glycol, Glycerol, Lactate, Isosorbide	Transportation, Housing, Safe Food Supply, Communication, Recreation,

The potential to convert these platform chemicals into industrial applicable chemicals is huge. A brief overview over the latter comprises: acrylates, acrylamides, 1,3-propanediol, 1,4-butanediol, tetrahydrofuran, γ-butyrolactone (GBL) and polymers like polyhydroxypolyamides. A demonstrative valuable application is the polymerization of acrylate and acrylamides, which can be produced via 3-hydroxypropionate (**Figure 1.1 A**). These compounds can be crosslinked to copolymers which have a very high water absorbency (Liu and Rempel, 1997). This technique is nowadays used in diapers and soft contact lenses. Furthermore, succinate, a metabolite of the tricarboxylic acid cycle in all organisms (Fernie et al., 2004), can be converted to commodity chemicals like tetrahydrofuran or γ-butyrolactone (GBL) (**Figure 1.1 B**). Notably, the latter has a broad application, in industry as plasticizer (McKinlay et al., 2007), as a valuable precursor for pharmaceuticals (Choi et al., 2013) or as a commonly known anaesthetic agent (Lenz et al., 2008).

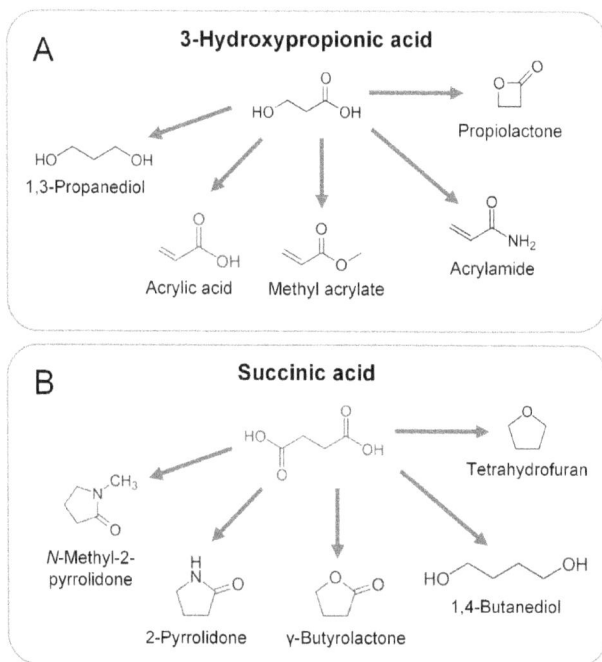

Figure 1.1. Overview of industrial important products derived from platform chemicals. The carbon-three compound 3-hydroxypropionate is used for the production of e.g. acrylates, which are processed to superabsorbent polymers among others (**A**). The carbon-four diacid succinate is processed into solvents, e.g. 1,4-butanediol or tetrahydrofuran (**B**).

1.2 Objectives

The objective of the present work was to broaden the use of *B. succiniciproducens* and derive carbon-three compounds. In particular, the heterologous production of L-alanine, β-alanine, and 3-hydroxypropionate from β-alanine, should be evaluated. Up to date, little is known about the ability of *B. succiniciproducens* to express heterologous genes, in particular suitable promoters, which can be deployed for achieving high expression levels. At first, enhancing the genetic toolbox was targeted. Therefore, set-up of a blue-white screening system in a *lacZ* deficient strain was done. Furthermore, suitable promoters for heterologous expression of various genes should be identified. The second step aimed at the utilization of appropriate genes and gene clusters for heterologous synthesis of the target products. Producing strains should then be developed and improved step-wise, using systems metabolic engineering. Finally, suitable process conditions for overproduction should be identified and applied.

2 THEORETICAL BACKGROUND

2.1 *Basfia succiniciproducens* – a novel industrial workhorse

The identification of succinate as a top value added chemical by the US DoE, initialized a rapid and parallelized run for commercialization of bio-based succinate. This led to the discovery of *B. succiniciproducens* DD1 (Kuhnert et al., 2010; Scholten and Dägele, 2008), isolated from the rumen of a Holstein cow (Kuhnert et al., 2010). Subsequent investigation generated succinate overproducers during the last decade (Becker et al., 2013; Lange et al., 2017; Scholten and Dägele, 2008; Scholten et al., 2009; Stellmacher et al., 2010). The microbe can utilize a variety of feed stocks (Kuhnert et al., 2010), including glycerol (Scholten and Dägele, 2008). Glycerol depicts a bulk by-product in biodiesel industry (Yang et al., 2012), make it a cheap and common used substrate.

Alongside, transcriptomics and fluxomics were used to elucidate its unexplored metabolism and identify targets for metabolic engineering (Becker et al., 2013; Scholten et al., 2009; Stellmacher et al., 2010). In particular, gene knockouts (Becker et al., 2013) or homologous gene expression (Lange et al., 2017) were investigated for succinate overproduction. Taken together, this provides a solid start point for further metabolic engineering of *B. succiniciproducens*.

2.1.1 The distinct metabolism and physiology of *Basfia succiniciproducens*

The first isolate of *B. succiniciproducens*, named DD1, was enriched from the bovine rumen of a Holstein cow, while screening for native succinate producers (Scholten and Dägele, 2008). Seven strains were isolated (Kuhnert et al., 2010) and taxonomically assigned to the family *Pasteurellaceae* by assessing the 16S rRNA, *rpoB*, *infB* and the *recN* gene sequences. Distinct phenotypical aspects of the *Pasteurellaceae* family include a capnophilic, facultative anaerobic, non-spore-forming, and non-motile lifestyle. The cells are gram-negative and coccoid to rod-shaped (Kuhnert et al., 2010). The *Pasteurellaceae* family comprises primary or opportunistic pathogens of the respiratory and genital tract of vertebrates (Dousse et al., 2008; Guettler et al., 1999). However, the isolated strain DD1 is neither toxic nor pathogenic against bovine, human or fish cell lines (Kuhnert et al., 2010). This is beneficial for development of industrial relevant processes, by reducing costs and handling risks. Additionally, only a few vitamins are essential for the strain (Hong et al., 2004), allowing minimal medium cultivation and consequently exact investigations of phenotypic aspects.

The genome sequence of *B. succiniciproducens* DD1 comprises 2.34 Mbp with 2363 open reading frames (ORFs) (Kuhnert et al., 2010). It is related (95 % on DNA and amino acid sequence level) to *Mannheimia succiniciproducens* MBEL55E, another prominent succinate producer (Lee et al., 2002). Of the 2380 ORFs found in the *M. succiniciproducens* genome, 2006 ORFs are homologous to *B. succiniciproducens* and might be regarded as a core genome (Kuhnert et al., 2010).

The central carbon metabolism of *B. succiniciproducens* DD1 (**Figure 2.1**) is composed by the Embden-Meyerhof-Parnas (EMP) pathway, and fueling the pentose phosphate (PP) pathway. Furthermore, the gluconeogenesis is found, which uses malic enzyme (*sfcA*), malate dehydrogenase (*mdh*), phosphoenolpyruvate carboxykinase (*pckA*) and fructose-1,6-bisphosphatase (*fbp*, *glpX*) to bypass the irreversible reactions of EMP pathway. The Entner-Doudoroff (ED) pathway, connected to gluconate metabolism, is found inactive (Becker et al., 2013). Several (carbohydrate) transporters, comprising phosphotransferase systems and ABC transporters, are annotated, which obviously mediated succinate production from different substrates (glycerol, sucrose, glucose, fructose, xylose, arabinose, galactose and mannose) (Scholten and Dägele, 2008). Due to its niche lifestyle in the bovine rumen, the observed efficient succinate formation from different feedstocks evolved by natural selection. The role of *B. succiniciproducens* in the bovine rumen is specialized as a part of the hosts microbial digestion, in a symbiotic manner. Its broad substrate spectrum enables conversion of plant carbohydrates from the bovine feed into succinate. Succinate is subsequently decarboxylated into propionate by the microbial rumen flora. The latter is then utilized by the host, underlining the importance of *B. succiniciproducens* as a member of the rumen flora (Guettler et al., 1999). Due to the specialized function of the rumen, the phenotypical succinate production is furthermore found in other rumen bacteria, e.g. *M. succiniciproducens* (Lee et al., 2002) and *Actinobacillus succinogenes* (Guettler et al., 1999). Additionally, acetate, formate and lactate and ethanol are the major and minor by-products of the metabolism, respectively (Becker et al., 2013).

Recently, metabolic flux analysis (Becker et al., 2013) allowed first insights into the specialized metabolism of *B. succiniciproducens*. High yield succinate production is mainly achieved through the reductive branch of the TCA cycle, whereas the contribution of the oxidative branch is negligible (**Figure 2.1**). The latter is a consequence of the beneficial incorporation of CO_2, while ATP is formed. This step is conducted by the anaplerotic ATP-dependent phosphoenolpyruvate carboxykinase (**Figure 2.1**), fueling the reductive branch of the TCA cycle (Becker et al., 2013). The enzyme links CO_2 incorporation to energy generation and cell growth. This was demonstrated by *pckA* knockout studies in *M. succiniciproducens* (Lee et al., 2006). As suggested for *M. succiniciproducens*, it appears likely that fumarate functions as an electron acceptor (Hong et al., 2004).

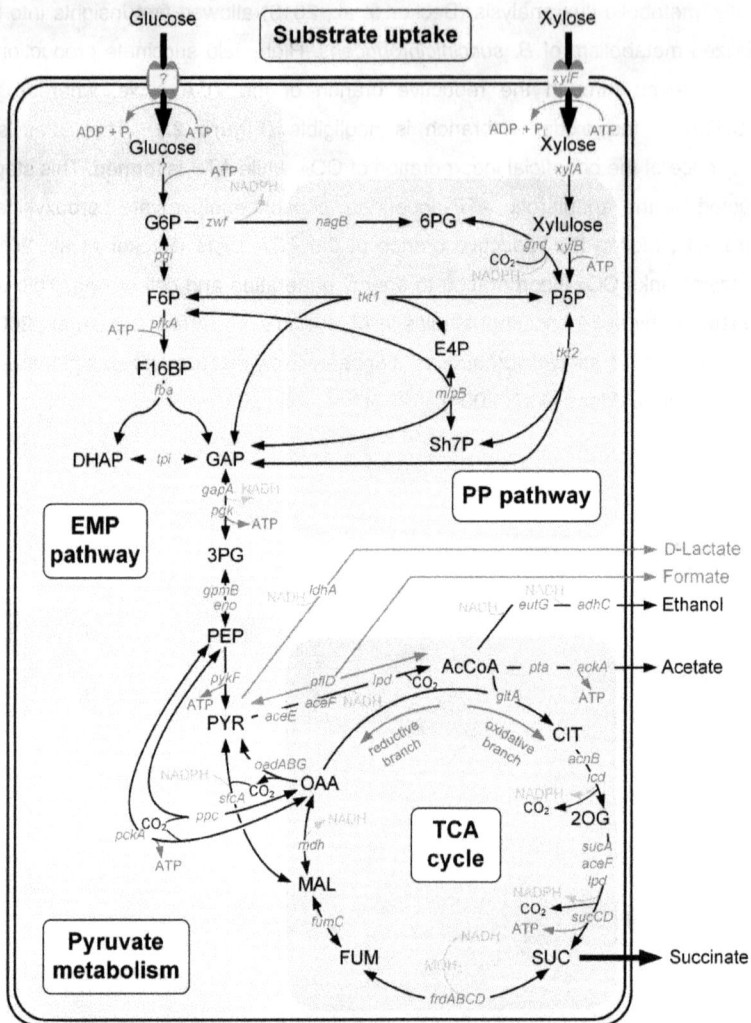

Figure 2.1. Central carbon metabolism of *B. succiniciproducens* DD1. Substrate carbon is taken up and channeled through the core metabolism by the EMP (glycolysis) and pentose phosphate (PP) pathway. Specific reactions at the pyruvate node and in the TCA cycle act reversible. The genes, encoding enzymes which catalyze the interconversions, are given in *italics*. Reactions corresponding to energy conversion are depicted in red, while redox reactions are indicated in orange. Gray arrows indicate reactions, which are eliminated in the used strain of the present study: *B. succiniciproducens* Δ*ldhA* Δ*pflD* (DD3). Question marks (?) denote unidentified genes. Abbreviations are: G6P, glucose 6-phosphate; 6PG, 6-phosphogluconate; P5P, pentose 5-phosphate; Sh7P, sedoheptulose 7-phosphate; E4P, erythrose 4-phosphate; F6P, fructose 6-phosphate; F16BP, fructose 1,6-bisphosphate; DHAP, dihydroxyacetone phosphate; GAP, glyceraldehyde 3-phosphate; 3PG, 3-phospho glycerate; PEP, phosphoenolpyruvate; PYR, pyruvate; OAA, oxaloacetate; AcCoA, acetyl-CoA; CIT, citrate; 2OG; 2-oxoglutarate; SUC, succinate; FUM, fumarate; MAL, malate; MQH$_2$, menaquinol; ATP, adenosine triphosphate; NADH, nicotineamide adenine dinucleotide, reduced; NADPH, nicotineamide adenine dinucleotide phosphate, reduced.

2.2 The C$_4$ platform chemical succinate – an industrial production accessible using *Basfia succiniciproducens*

Since biotechnological production of acetate and citrate, back in 1823 (Raspor and Goranovič, 2008) and 1913 (Zahorski, 1913), organic acids belong to the veterans of bio-based goods (Alonso et al., 2014; Becker et al., 2015). Beyond traditional uses in feed and food, particularly the renaissance of bio-plastics has pushed bio-production of organic acids as bi-functional monomers. Acids with additional keto- or hydroxyl-groups are desirable building blocks for polyesters, and di-carboxylic acids are used for the production of polyamides with advanced material properties (Becker and Wittmann, 2015). Recently, succinate, an intermediate of the tricarboxylic acid (TCA) cycle, evoked a strong research interest for its bio-based production. This carbon-four 1,4-diacid provides a basic chemistry, similar to the petrochemically derived maleic acid/anhydride, which is beneficial for manufacturing biopolymers or solvents like butanediol, maleic anhydride and nylon-type polymers (Beauprez et al., 2010; Becker et al., 2015; Werpy et al., 2004).

Beside the biotechnology workhorses *Escherichia coli* and *Corynebacterium glutamicum*, members of the *Pasteurellaceae* family appeared promising for succinate production (Guettler et al., 1999; Lee et al., 2002; Scholten and Dägele, 2008). *A. succinogenes* (Pateraki et al., 2016), *M. succiniciproducens* (Kim et al., 2017) and *B. succiniciproducens* (Becker et al., 2013; Cimini et al., 2016) revealed their potential in bio-based succinate production. These bacteria are to date well-established industrial bio-succinate producers with a broader substrate spectrum (Dousse et al., 2008; Guettler et al., 1999; Kim et al., 2004; Scholten and Dägele, 2008).

The intensive research in this field contributed to our current understanding of microbial succinate fermentation and its optimization (Becker et al., 2015). In brief, reviewed rational strategies exploited the elimination of by-product formation (Becker et al., 2013; Cheng et al., 2013; Litsanov et al., 2012) and amplification of the anaplerotic flux toward the reductive TCA cycle branch (Cheng et al., 2013; Litsanov et al., 2012). Additionally, renewable substrates like lignocellulosic derived xylose (Salvachúa et al., 2016) and sucrose (Lange et al., 2017) were considered, recently.

9

As example, Lange et al. (2017) demonstrated the powerful use of ^{13}C metabolic flux analysis for metabolic engineering of *B. succiniciproducens* for efficient sucrose utilization. The overexpression of a newly discovered fructokinase (*rbsK*), the deletion of the competing fructose PTS and the combination of both strategies led to synergistic improvements in succinate production from sucrose. It was demonstrated, that *B. succiniciproducens* DD1 Δ*fruA*, lacking the fructose PTS, produced 71 g L^{-1} succinate at a yield of 2.5 mol mol^{-1}. Apparently, a 12 % improvement of the succinate titer was achieved, compared to the parent strain *B. succiniciproducens* DD1. An overview of the most relevant native and recombinant microbial succinate production hosts is given in **Table 2.1**.

Table 2.1. Succinate production performance of native and recombinant microbial production hosts.

Organism	Substrate	Process operation	Max. titer [g L^{-1}]	Max. yield [g g^{-1}]	Max. STY[a] [g L^{-1} h^{-1}]	Reference
Corynebacterium glutamicum Δ*ldhA*-pCRA717	Glucose	Dual phase fed-batch	146.0	0.92	3.17	(Okino et al., 2008)
Corynebacterium glutamicum BOL-3/pAN6-*gap*	Glucose and formate	Dual phase fed-batch	134.0	1.09	2.53	(Litsanov et al., 2012)
Escherichia coli NZN111 Δ*pflB*Δ*ldhA*	Cassava starch	Dual phase fed-batch	127.0	0.86	3.23	(Chen et al., 2014)
Actinobacillus succinogenes 130Z[T]	Glucose	Batch	106.0	0.80	1.34	(Guettler et al., 1996)
Escherichia coli AFP111-*pyc*	Glucose	Dual phase batch	99.2	1.10	1.30	(Vemuri et al., 2002)
Basfia succiniciproducens Δ*fruA*	Sucrose	Fed-batch	71.0	0.84	3.13[b]	(Lange et al., 2017)
Mannheimia succiniciproducens Δ*ldh*Δ*pfl*Δ*pta*Δ*ack*	Glucose	Fed-batch	52.4	0.76	1.80	(Cheng et al., 2013)
Basfia succiniciproducens DD1 Δ*ldhA*Δ*pflD*	Glucose	Batch	31.7	0.71	1.50	(Becker et al., 2013; Scholten and Dägele, 2008; Stellmacher et al., 2010)
Basfia succiniciproducens CCUG 57335	DDAPH[c]	Batch	30.6	0.69	1.05[b]	(Salvachúa et al., 2016)
Basfia succiniciproducens DD1	Glycerol	Batch	8.4	1.20	0.90	(Scholten and Dägele, 2008)

[a] STY = Space Time Yield
[b] estimated from reference
[c] DDAPH is defined as high xylose-content hydrolysate from corn stover (see reference)

More recently, the commercialization of bio-succinate was achieved by four companies, namely BioAmber (Canada), Myriant (USA), Succinity (Germany) and Reverdia (The Netherlands) (**Table 2.2**).

The Succinity process relies on *B. succiniciproducens*. Up to date, 10,000 tons per annum are produced at a production site located in Spain (Becker et al., 2015). Myriant uses an engineered *E. coli* strain. Succinate production by BioAmber and Reverdia, a joint venture of DSM and Roquette, is driven in large scale, using *Candida krusei* and *Saccharomyces cerevisiae*, respectively (Jansen and van Gulik, 2014). The use of yeasts allows lower pH values, advantageous for economic recovery of succinic acid during downstream processing (Yan et al., 2014). In addition, evolutionary adaptation was successfully applied to enhance production and tolerance (Jiang et al., 2014; Kwon et al., 2011; Li et al., 2013). As example, engineered strains of *E. coli* and *C. glutamicum* reach high-level production of up to 127 g L^{-1} and 146 g L^{-1} succinate, respectively (Becker and Wittmann, 2015). In addition to anaerobic succinate fermentation, aerobic processes are currently evaluated. This was shown by a proprietary Royal DSM yeast strain, producing 43 g L^{-1} succinate with a yield of 0.45 g g^{-1} on glucose (Cheng et al., 2013).

Table 2.2. **Industrial succinate production of organic acid from biomass feedstocks.** The data is derived from (Becker et al., 2015).

Company	Annual production capacity (plant site) [t a^{-1}]	Organism	Feedstock
Succinity[a]	10,000 (Spain)	*Basfia succiniciproducens*	Glycerol, sugars
Myriant[b]	13,600 (USA)	*Escherichia coli*	Sorghum
BioAmber[c]	3000 (France, demonstration plant)	*Escherichia coli*, yeast (possibly *Candida krusei*)	Corn
Reverdia[d]	10,000 (Italy)	Low pH yeast (*Saccharomyces cerevisiae*)	Starch

[a] Joint venture between BASF SE and Corbion Purac.
[b] Cooperation with ThyssenKrupp Uhde.
[c] Joint venture between DNP Green Technology, ARD, and Mitsui & Co.
[d] Joint venture between Royal DSM N.V. and Roquette Frères.

2.3 C₃ chemicals – industrial chemicals of interest to be derived by *Basfia succiniciproducens*

2.3.1 Pyruvate

When organic carbon-three acids are mentioned, pyruvate is one of the commonly known products. Especially, pyruvate is not only a central key intermediate of microbial, plant, animal and human metabolism, but also a chemical precursor for various derivatives and polymers, and an ingredient of diverse commodity products (Wieschalka et al., 2013). As chemical production is not very cost efficient, bio-based production through fermentation got in focus.

In order to achieve pyruvate production, the diverse catabolic and anabolic pathways as well as fermentation routes, competing with pyruvate formation, have to be considered. The elimination of such reactions, for example lactate dehydrogenase, pyruvate dehydrogenase, pyruvate-formate lyase, pyruvate oxidase and pyruvate decarboxylase is thus of major interest (Li et al., 2001). Since pyruvate is generated in the EMP pathway (or the ED pathway), the increased supply of the needed co-factors, such as NAD^+ and ADP, is desired (Maleki and Eiteman, 2017). Bio-based production has been established using multi-auxotrophic yeast and *E. coli* (Becker et al., 2015; Maleki and Eiteman, 2017). By now, the highest titers have been obtained for *E. coli* (90 g L^{-1}) (Zhu et al., 2008) and *S. cerevisiae* (135 g L^{-1}) (van Maris et al., 2004), though other producers are being developed (**Table 2.3**).

2.3.2 Lactate

In contrast, production of lactate, a derivative of pyruvate, is an established business in biotechnology with NatureWorks (USA), Purac (The Netherlands), Galactic (Belgium) and several Chinese companies as major suppliers of around 400,000 tons lactate annually (Choi et al., 2015).

Metabolically, lactate is a direct product of D/L-lactate dehydrogenase, which reduces pyruvate to the corresponding enantiomer of lactate. Current processes are operated with classically optimized Lactobacilli (Becker and Wittmann, 2015) and engineered yeast (**Table 2.3**), whereby also other producers exhibit excellent performance (Xu and Xu, 2014; Yamane and Tanaka, 2013). As example, immobilized mycelia of *Rhizopus oryzae* even surpass 230 g L^{-1} lactate, the highest titer reported so far

(Yamane and Tanaka, 2013). In addition, metabolic engineering has generated other potent production strains, which are particularly useful to obtain the optically pure product. Highly pure L-lactate production could be realized using *E. coli* (138 g L^{-1}) and *S. cerevisiae* (122 g L^{-1}), while *C. glutamicum* was successfully trained for D-lactate production (**Table 2.3**). A remarkable high titer of 195 g L^{-1} D-lactate was achieved by a synergistic amplified expression of five glycolytic genes, namely glucokinase (GLK), glyceraldehyde 3-phosphate dehydrogenase (GAPDH), phosphofructokinase (PFK), triosephosphate isomerase (TPI) and bisphosphate aldolase (FBA) with PFK as one of the key reactions (Tsuge et al., 2015). Future improvements can be expected from recent research on cellular energetics, alternative substrates (Buschke et al., 2013) and photoautotrophic production from CO_2 using cyanobacteria (Li et al., 2015).

2.3.3 L-Alanine

With a world market of more than four million tons per year, amino acids are among the most important products in industrial biotechnology (Becker and Wittmann, 2012b). Almost all amino acids are exclusively derived by microbial fermentation, because this provides the biologically active L-enantiomer. The biosynthesis of amino acids is hereby closely linked to central metabolism via the supply of carbon building blocks, nitrogen, reducing power and energy. This poses complex demands on the producing cell. The L-alanine depicts one of the smallest chiral compounds (Zhou et al., 2015) used in food and pharmaceutical applications. Compared to the market size of lysine (1.5 mio t a^{-1}) (Becker and Wittmann, 2015), L-alanine production is rather small, estimated to be about 500 t a^{-1}, limited by its high production costs (Zhang et al., 2007). This can be overcome by recently established basic producers (Becker and Wittmann, 2015).

As lactate, alanine can be derived from pyruvate by use of an alanine dehydrogenase (Zhang et al., 2007). Additionally, aspartate decarboxylases exist, producing L-alanine by decarboxylation of L-aspartate. Surplus, L-alanine is produced in many transamination reactions (Oikawa, 2007). Current processes rely on expression of alanine dehydrogenases from *Geobacillus stearothermophilus* in *E. coli* (Zhang et al., 2007; Zhou et al., 2015) or *Lysinibacillus sphaericus* in *C. glutamicum* (Jojima et al., 2010; Yamamoto et al., 2012) (**Table 2.3**). The highest titer reported so far, was reached by *C. glutamicum* (216 g L^{-1}) (Yamamoto et al., 2012). Using *E. coli*, 121 g L^{-1} with outstanding volumetric productivities (4.18 g L^{-1} h^{-1}) in an oxygen-limited process were obtained (Zhou et al., 2015). A new player in the field is the recently evoked marine organism *Vibrio natriegens* (Lee et al., 2016; Weinstock et al., 2016), which was lately engineered for alanine production. This fast-growing organism demonstrated a highly outstanding volumetric productivity of 0.56 g alanine L^{-1} min^{-1} (34 g L^{-1} h^{-1}) under anaerobic conditions due to its high specific glucose uptake rates (7.8 g g^{-1} h^{-1}) (Hoffart et al., 2017).

2.3.4 β-Alanine

An achiral isomer of alanine, containing the amino group in β-position, is commonly known as β-alanine or 3-aminopropionate (Liang et al., 2008). This special amino acid is used for an increasing number of applications, concerning production of important nitrogen-containing chemicals (Song et al., 2015) and athlete nutrition (Nassis et al., 2017). Moreover, this compound plays a somewhat essential role in synthesis of the vitamin pantothenate. Here, two metabolic pathways are connected by the pantothenate synthase which condenses pantoate with β-alanine to form pantothenate (Dusch et al., 1999). Commonly, β-alanine is synthesized by a pyruvoyl-dependent protein, *panD*, which is found in many organisms, e.g. *E. coli* and *C. glutamicum* (Dusch et al., 1999; Stuecker et al., 2012). This aspartate 1-decarboxylase is expressed as a pre-protein and then cleaved to yield the active pro-protein form.

A lately published study brought evidence, that a protein family, named *panP*, provides also aspartate 1-decarboxylase activity, but is suggested to be pyridoxal-dependent (Pan et al., 2017).

Commonly, biological production of β-alanine was performed using β-aminopropionitrile as substrate in whole-cell bioconversions of *Alcaligenes* sp. OMT-MY14, *Aminobacter aminobrance* ATCC 23314 (Song et al., 2015) and *Rhodococcus* sp. G20 (Liang et al., 2008). Also, *panD* based whole-cell or enzymatic L-aspartate conversion is described in literature (Konst et al., 2009; Shen et al., 2014). Recently, an aerobic fermentation process was presented, allowing the production of 32 g L^{-1} β-alanine from glucose, using an engineered *E. coli* strain expressing the *panD* gene from *C. glutamicum* (Song et al., 2015). This depicts a valuable study of bio-based recombinant β-alanine synthesis from sugars (**Table 2.3**).

2.3.5 3-Hydroxypropionate (3-HP)

Since biotechnological production of lactate is commonly established, bio-based production of its isomer 3-hydroxypropionate was focused in the last years. As one of the top-value chemicals from biomass, 3-HP was identified due to its huge market potential as chemical precursor for acrylic acid (Werpy et al., 2004). In brief, commercial interesting commodity and specialty chemicals like 1,3-propanediol, acrylate, methyl acrylate and acrylamide, with significant market opportunities, can be derived from 3-HP (Werpy et al., 2004).

Since then, chemical companies involving BASF (Germany), Cargill (USA), Dow Chemical (USA) and Novozymes (Denmark) are chasing for commercialization of a bio-based production process (Choi et al., 2015). Indeed, the portfolio of potential pathways for fermentative 3-HP production is rather broad (Valdehuesa et al., 2013), being chance and challenge at the same time. The most straightforward bio-based route relies on glycerol utilization only requiring two enzymes, namely glycerol dehydratase and aldehyde dehydrogenase. Consequently, this approach yielded the best processes so far, using *E. coli* and *Klebsiella pneumoniae* as production hosts (**Table 2.3**) with high conversion yields of up to 0.88 g g^{-1} for *E. coli* (Kim et al., 2014). Discrete substrate feeding of glucose and glycerol for growth and production, respectively, boosted product titer to 72 g L^{-1} (Chu et al., 2015). Glucose-based production has been developed through implementation of the malonyl-CoA and the β-alanine route toward 3-HP in *E. coli* (Rathnasingh et al., 2009; Song et al., 2016) reaching 38.7 g L^{-1} and 31 g L^{-1} 3-HP, respectively. The β-alanine route was also implemented in *S. cerevisiae*, demonstrating the production of 13.7 g L^{-1} 3-HP (Borodina et al., 2015). These studies relied on a discrete set of enzymatic reactions using acetyl-CoA (malonyl-CoA route) and oxaloacetate (β-alanine route) as precursors.

Only recently, Cargill has acquired a proprietary glucose-based fermentation process with recombinant *E. coli*, capable of producing approximately 50 g L^{-1} 3-HP with a yield of 0.53 g g^{-1}, which was initially patented by the US company OPXbio (Lynch et al., 2015).

Table 2.3. Production performance of recombinant microbial production hosts of organic acids.

Product	Organism	Substrate	Process operation	Max. titer [g L^{-1}]	Max. yield [g g^{-1}]	Max. STY[a] [g L^{-1} h^{-1}]	Ref.
Pyruvate	S. cerevisiae	Glucose	Fed-batch	135	0.54	1.35[b]	(van Maris et al., 2004)
	E. coli	Glucose	Fed-batch	90	0.68	2.10	(Zhu et al., 2008)
	C. glutamicum	Glucose	Fed-batch	44	0.47	0.44[b]	(Wieschalka et al., 2013)
D-/L-Lactate	R. oryzae	Glucose	Fed-batch, immobilized mycelia	231	0.93[b]	1.83	(Yamane and Tanaka, 2013)
	C. glutamicum	Glucose	Fed-batch	195	0.90	6.10[b]	(Tsuge et al., 2015)
	B. coagulans	Cane molasses	Fed-batch	168	0.88	2.10	(Xu and Xu, 2014)
	E. coli	Glucose	Fed-batch	138	0.99	6.30	(Becker and Wittmann, 2015)
	S. cerevisiae	Glucose	Batch	122	-	2.50[b]	(Becker and Wittmann, 2015)
	C. glutamicum	Glucose	Fed-batch	120	-	4.00[b]	(Becker and Wittmann, 2012a)
L-Alanine	C. glutamicum	Glucose	Batch	216	0.92	4.50[b]	(Yamamoto et al., 2012)
	E. coli	Glucose	Fed-batch	121	0.96	4.18	(Zhou et al., 2015)
	E. coli	Glucose	Batch	114	0.95	4.04	(Zhang et al., 2007)
	C. glutamicum	Glucose	Fed-batch	98	0.83	3.10	(Jojima et al., 2010)
	V. natriegens	Glucose	Batch	34[b]	0.81	34.00	(Hoffart et al., 2017)
β-Alanine	E. coli	Glucose	Fed-batch	32	0.14	0.83	(Song et al., 2015)
	PanD$_{cgl}$ enzyme	Aspartate	pH-stat, fed-batch	12.9	0.97	0.36[b]	(Shen et al., 2014)
	R. sp. G20	β-amino-propionitrile	Batch	8.9[b]	0.99[b]	6.7[b]	(Liang et al., 2008)
3-HP	E. coli	Glucose Glycerol	Fed-batch	72	-	1.80	(Chu et al., 2015)
	E. coli	Glycerol	Fed-batch	57	0.88	1.59	(Kim et al., 2014)
	K. pneumoniae	Glycerol	Fed-batch	49	0.40[b]	1.75[b]	(Huang et al., 2013)
	E. coli	Glucose	Fed-batch	48	0.53	-	(Lynch et al., 2015)
	S. cerevisiae	Glucose	Fed-batch	14	0.07[b]	0.17[b]	(Borodina et al., 2015)

[a] STY = Space Time Yield
[b] Estimated from reference

3 MATERIAL AND METHODS

3.1 Bacterial strains and plasmids

For cloning purposes, *E. coli* TOP10 (Invitrogen, Darmstadt, Germany) was used. *B. succiniciproducens* Δ*ldhA* Δ*pflD* (DD3) and *B. succiniciproducens* ALA-1 was obtained from previous work (Becker et al., 2013; Fabarius, 2013). Transformation of *B. succiniciproducens* was performed, using the episomal *Pasteurellaceae* vector pJFF224-XN (Frey, 1992) and the integrative vector pClik^{CM}, respectively (Becker et al., 2013). *B. succiniciproducens* DD3Δ*DD0759*Δ*DD0810*, lacking the native *lacZ* genes *DD0810* and *DD0759*, was constructed by Nadja Barton (Institute of Systems Biotechnology, Saarland University) during her master thesis (Barton, 2015). All strains and plasmids used in this work are listed in **Table 3.1**.

3.2 Genes used for metabolic engineering

The native aspartate 1-decarboxylase from *E. coli* K12 MG1655 (*panD$_{eco}$*, KEGG entry: b0131), *C. glutamicum* ATCC13032 (*panD$_{cgl}$*, KEGG entry: Cgl0135) and *Vibrio natriegens* DSM759 (*panP$_{vna}$*, KEGG entry: PN96_07390) were used. Furthermore, the β-alanine-pyruvate transaminase from *P. putida* KT2440 (*bapta$_{ppu}$*, KEGG entry: PP_0596) and the malonic semialdehyde reductase from *E. coli* K12 MG1655 (*ydfG$_{eco}$*, KEGG entry: ydfG) were codon-optimized (**Table 6.2**) on DNA level for stable expression in *B. succiniciproducens* (Thermo Fisher Scientific, Regensburg, Germany). All used genes and their specific functions are summarized in **Table 3.2**.

MATERIAL AND METHODS

Table 3.1. Bacterial strains and plasmids.

Strain	Description	Source and reference
E. coli TOP10 / DH10B	Cloning host	Invitrogen, Darmstadt, Germany
B. succiniciproducens DD3	$\Delta ldhA$ $\Delta pflD$	(Becker *et al.*, 2013)
DD3$\Delta\Delta lacZ$	$\Delta lacZ$-DD0759 $\Delta lacZ$-DD0810	This study
DD3$\Delta\Delta lacZ\Delta DD0789$-neo	$\Delta lacZ$-DD0759 $\Delta lacZ$-DD0810 $\Delta DD0789$::$P_{neo}neo$	This study
DD3 ALA-1	$alaD\_gstear$::$pflD$	(Fabarius, 2013)
DD3 + pJFF224	pJFF224-XN	This study
DD3 + Bsuc_PL8	$P_{pflD}GFP$	This study
DD3 + Bsuc_PL9	$P_{pflA}GFP$	This study
DD3 + Bsuc_PL10	$P_{ldhA}GFP$	This study
DD3 + Bsuc_PL11	$P_{sodc}GFP$	This study
DD3 + Bsuc_PL25	$P_{pflD}panD_{eco}$	This study
DD3 + Bsuc_PL26	$P_{pflD}panD_{cgl}$	This study
DD3 + Bsuc_PL47	$P_{EM7*}panD_{cgl}$	This study
DD3 + Bsuc_PL80	$P_{EM7*}panD^+_{cgl}$	This study
DD3 + Bsuc_PL86	$P_{pflD}panD^+_{cgl}$	This study
DD3 + Bsuc_PL105	$P_{EM7*}PN96\_07390_{vna}$ ($panP_{vna}$)	This study
DD3 + Bsuc_PL27	$P_{pflD}bapta_{ppu}{}^+$-$P_{pflD}ydfG_{eco}{}^+$	This study
DD3 + Bsuc_PL52	$P_{EM7*}panD_{cgl}$-RBS_{EM7*}-$bapta_{ppu}{}^+$-RBS_{EM7*}-$ydfG_{eco}$	This study
DD3 + Bsuc_PL98	$P_{EM7*}panD_{cgl}{}^+$-RBS_{EM7*}-$bapta_{ppu}{}^+$-RBS_{EM7*}-$ydfG_{eco}{}^+$	This study
DD3$\Delta\Delta lacZ$ + Bsuc_PL18	Complementation of *lacZ*-DD0810 by Bsuc_PL18	This study
DD3$\Delta\Delta lacZ$ + Bsuc_PL19	Complementation of *lacZ*-DD0759 by Bsuc_PL19	This study
Plasmids		
pJFF224-XN	XN cloning site, CM^R, mob oriV, RSF1010 replicon	(Frey, 1992)
pClik^{CM}	CM^R, $P_{sacB\text{-}sacB}$, ori-EC(pMB)	(Becker et al., 2013)
Bsuc_PL8	pJFF224 derivative, $P_{pflD}GFP$	This study
Bsuc_PL9	pJFF224 derivative, $P_{pflA}GFP$	This study
Bsuc_PL10	pJFF224 derivative, $P_{ldhA}GFP$	This study
Bsuc_PL11	pJFF224 derivative, $P_{sodc}GFP$	This study
Bsuc_PL104	pJFF224 derivative, $P_{EM7*}GFP$	This study
Bsuc_PL25	pJFF224 derivative, ($P_{pflD}panD_{eco}$)	This study
Bsuc_PL26	pJFF224 derivative, ($P_{pflD}panD_{cgl}$)	This study
Bsuc_PL47	pJFF224 derivative, ($P_{EM7*}panD_{cgl}$)	This study
Bsuc_PL80	pJFF224 derivative, ($P_{EM7*}panD_{cgl}{}^*$)	This study
Bsuc_PL86	pJFF224 derivative, ($P_{pflD}panD_{cgl}{}^*$)	This study
Bsuc_PL105	pJFF224 derivative, ($P_{EM7*}PN96\_07390_{vna}$)	This study
Bsuc_PL27	pJFF224 derivative, ($P_{pflD}bapta_{ppu}{}^+$-$P_{pflD}ydfG_{eco}{}^+$)	This study
Bsuc_PL52	pJFF224 derivative, ($P_{EM7*}panD_{cgl}$-RBS_{EM7*}-$bapta_{ppu}{}^+$-RBS_{EM7*}-$ydfG_{eco}{}^+$	This study
Bsuc_PL98	pJFF224 derivative, ($P_{EM7*}panD_{cgl}{}^*$-RBS_{EM7*}-$bapta_{ppu}{}^+$-RBS_{EM7*}-$ydfG_{eco}{}^+$)	This study
Bsuc_PL16	pClik^{CM} derivative, $\Delta lacZ$-DD0810	This study
Bsuc_PL17	pClik^{CM} derivative, $\Delta lacZ$-DD0759	This study
Bsuc_PL87	pClik^{CM} derivative, 200 bp US-*lacZ*-DD0759-*lacZ*-DD0759	This study
Bsuc_PL88	pClik^{CM} derivative, 200 bp US-*lacY*-DD0811-RBS_{DD0810}-*lacZ*-DD0810	This study
Bsuc_PL18	pJFF224 derivative, 200 bp US-*lacY*-DD0811-RBS_{DD0810}-*lacZ*-DD0810	This study
Bsuc_PL19	pJFF224 derivative, 200 bp US-*lacZ*-DD0759-*lacZ*-DD0759	This study
Bsuc_PL94	Bsuc_PL87 de., $\Delta DD0789$-sucrose PTS::$P_{neo}neo$	This study
Bsuc_PL95	Bsuc_PL88 de., $\Delta DD0789$-sucrose PTS::$P_{neo}neo$	This study

$^+$ Genes are codon-optimized for *B. succiniciproducens*
* P_{EM7*} mutated version of P_{EM7} and its ribosomal binding site (RBS) from a *P. putida* specific project (Rogsch, 2015)
de. = derivative

Table 3.2. Genes used for metabolic engineering.

Gene	KEGG entry	Enzyme	Function	Codon optimization
$panD_{eco}$ (E. coli)	b0131	Aspartate 1-decarboxylase		-
$panD_{cgl}$ (C. glutamicum)	Cgl0135	Aspartate 1-decarboxylase		-
$panD_{eco}^+$ (E. coli)	b0131	Aspartate 1-decarboxylase	β-Alanine synthesis	+
$panD_{cgl}^+$ (C. glutamicum)	Cgl0135	Aspartate 1-decarboxylase		+
$panP_{vna}$ (V. natriegens)	PN96_07390	Aspartate 1-decarboxylase		-
$bapta_{ppu}^+$ (P. putida)	PP_0596	β-Alanine-pyruvate transaminase	Malonate semialdehyde synthesis	+
$ydfG_{eco}^+$ (E. coli)	ydfG	Malonic semialdehyde reductase	3-HP synthesis	+

3.3 Chemicals and media

3.3.1 Chemicals

Chemicals were of analytical grade and were derived from Sigma Aldrich (Taufkirchen, Germany), Roth (Karlsruhe, Germany), Merck (Darmstadt, Germany), and Becton Dickinson (Franklin Lakes, NJ, US), respectively, if not stated otherwise. Silylation reagents for gas chromatography were obtained from Macherey-Nagel (Düren, Germany). For qualitative labeling experiments, [$^{13}C_6$] glucose (99 % purity) and [$^{13}C_3{}^{15}N$] β-alanine (99 % purity), was obtained from Euriso-top (Saarbrücken, Germany) and Sigma Aldrich (Taufkirchen, Germany), respectively.

3.3.2 Media for genetic engineering

Strains of E. coli were maintained, using Luria Bertani broth (Becton Dickinson, Franklin Lakes, NJ, US) in liquid (LB Lennox) or in solid form (35 g L^{-1}, LB Lennox agar). For standard strain maintenance, genetic engineering and promoter screening of B. succiniciproducens, brain heart infusion (BHI) medium (Becton Dickinson, Franklin Lakes, NJ, US) was used (37 g L^{-1}). BHI solid medium was prepared, adding 18 g L^{-1} agar (Difco, Becton Dickinson, Franklin Lakes, NJ, US) and a combination of 9.38 g L^{-1} (N-morpholino)propanesulfonic acid (MOPS), 1.25 g L^{-1} Mg(OH)$_2$, 5.8 g L^{-1} 2,2-Bis(hydroxymethyl)-2,2',2"nitrilotriethanol (Bis-Tris), and 1.8 g L^{-1} NaHCO$_3$ as a buffer system. For selection of mutant strains with chloramphenicol resistance, 10 µg mL^{-1} (E. coli) or 5 µg mL^{-1} (B. succiniciproducens) of a chloramphenicol stock solution (50 mg mL^{-1} in ethanol) was added, respectively (**Table 6.1**).

3.3.3 Cultivation media

Media for aerobic or anaerobic cultivation of *B. succiniciproducens* were freshly prepared from sterile stock solutions and sterile demineralized water. An overview of the stock solutions is given in **Table 6.1**. Stock solutions containing glycine-betaine, trace elements (Young Lee, 1996), and vitamins (Becker et al., 2013) were stored at 4 °C prior to use for up to two weeks.

For aerobic cultivation, the first pre-culture was grown in BHI medium. The second pre-culture and the main-culture were carried out in triplicates in a complex medium described in **Table 3.3**. For each experiment, the medium was freshly prepared from the sterilized stock solutions (See appendix).

Minimal medium (**Table 3.4**) pre-cultures in 10 mL scale for anaerobic cultivation were inoculated directly with living cells from agar plates. All main-cultures were carried out as well in minimal medium in triplicates. The medium was freshly prepared from the sterilized stock solutions for each experiment (see appendix **Table 6.1**).

Table 3.3. Composition of complex medium for aerobic cultivation. The medium was freshly prepared from the sterile stock solutions. For certain experiments the specified carbon source stock solution was added to the medium.

Stock solution	Volume [mL]	Media concentration [g L⁻¹]
Glucose, 50 %	3.0	15
or Xylose, 50 %	3.0	15
or Sucrose, 50 %	3.0	15
or Fructose, 50 %	3.0	15
or Glycerol, 50 %	3.0	15
Yeast extract[a], 10 %	5.0	5
BHI[a], 10 %	5.0	5
Ammonium sulphate, 50%, pH 7.2	2.0	10
ACES, 500 mM, pH 7.2	40.0	200 mM
Sodium carbonate, 25 %	0.4	1
Phosphate, 50 %	0.6	3
Glycine-betaine, 500 mM	0.5	0.29
Salt solution, 14 %	1.0	1.4 %
Vitamin stock 1, 100x, pH 7.5	1.0	1x
Trace elements, 200x	0.5	1x
H₂O, demineralized	ad 100 mL	

[a] Becton and Dickinson

Table 3.4. Composition of minimal medium for anaerobic cultivation. The medium was freshly prepared from the sterile stock solutions. In the experiments, different carbon sources or L-aspartate/β-alanine were added to the medium as described below in detail. Chloramphenicol was added to maintain the episomal plasmid of *B. succiniciproducens* mutant strains. As an insoluble buffer system, MgCO₃ (30 g L⁻¹) was used, which was added right before autoclaving.

Stock solution	Volume [mL]	Media concentration [g L⁻¹]
Glucose, 50 %	6.0	30.0
or Xylose, 50 %	6.0	30.0
or Sucrose, 50 %	6.0	30.0
or Fructose, 50 %	6.0	30.0
or Glycerol, 50 %	6.0	30.0
L-Aspartate, 25 %[a]	2.0	5
β-Alanine, 25 %[a]	2.0	5
3-HP, 25 %[a]	2.0	5
Yeast extract[b,c], 10 %	0.1	0.1
Ammonium sulphate[d], 50 %	0.8 / 0.4	4.0 / 2.0
Phosphate, 50 %	0.6	3.0
Salt solution, 14 %	1.0	1.4
Vitamin stock 1, 100x, pH 7.5	1.0	
Chloramphenicol, 5 %	0.1	5 µg mL⁻¹
H₂O, demineralized	ad 100 mL	

[a] L-aspartate, β-alanine and 3-hydroxypropionate were supplied in certain experiments to support production of β-alanine or 3-hydroxypropionate or examine the metabolism, respectively
[b] Becton and Dickinson
[c] Yeast extract was added to minimal medium to support growth of *B. succiniciproducens* mutant strains
[d] β-alanine / 3-hydroxypropionate production was realized using 4 g L⁻¹ / 2 g L⁻¹ of Ammonium sulphate

3.4 Genetic engineering

Molecular methods and genetic engineering of *B. succiniciproducens* were based on standard protocols (Becker et al., 2013; Gibson et al., 2009; Mullis et al., 1986; Sambrook, 2001). The oligonucleotides used for plasmid construction and screening are listed in **Table 3.5**.

3.4.1 Isolation of nucleic acids

The isolation of purified genomic DNA was performed with the GeneElute™ Kit (Sigma Aldrich, Taufkirchen, Germany) as given by the manufacturer. Elution of purified DNA from preparation columns was performed with sterile demineralized water. Subsequently, the DNA concentration was measured, using the NanoDrop® Spectrophotometer ND-1000 (Thermo Fisher Scientific, Waltham, MA, USA).

Plasmid isolation from the cloning host *E. coli* TOP10 was conducted using the QIAprep Spin Miniprep Kit (Qiagen, Hilden, Germany). Plasmid DNA elution from columns was conducted using sterile demineralized water, pre-warmed at 65 °C.

Purification of amplified DNA from PCR mixtures or agarose gel suspensions was performed using the Wizard® SV Gel and PCR Clean-Up System (Promega, Fitchburg, WI, USA). Again, sterile demineralized water, pre-warmed at 65 °C, was used for elution.

Table 3.5. **Oligonucleotides used as primers for genetic engineering of *B. succiniciproducens* and plasmid or strain validation.** Gibson's Assembly primer overhangs are underlined. Restriction sites used for restriction-digestion based cloning are given bold in the sequence and defined in the table. Ribosome binding sites are underlined in bold and defined in the table. The specific target plasmid and the resulting amplicon is also given in the table.

#	5'-Sequence-3'	Site	Plasmid and amplicon
1	GCGGTGGCGGCCGCTCTAGAAATTTAGATATGTACCATTTAGTAATTA	-	Bsuc_PL8
2	TTCGAACTAGTTTGGACCATTTTTAATACTTCCTTCTTTTCTAGT	-	P$_{pflD}$
3	GAAAAGAAGGAAGTATTAAAAATGGTCCAAACTAGTTCGAA	-	Bsuc_PL8
4	TCTACTGGGGATCCGGGCCCTTATTTGTAGAGCTCATCCAT	-	GFP
5	GCGGTGGCGGCCGCTCTAGAACAATCAATGTAATTGAGAGTTTG	-	Bsuc_PL9
6	TTCGAACTAGTTTGGACCATAATATGCCCTTAAATAATCAACAAA	-	P$_{pflA}$
7	TGATTATTTAAGGGCATATTATGGTCCAAACTAGTTCGAA + 4	-	Bsuc_PL9 / GFP
8	GCGGTGGCGGCCGCTCTAGACCGAACTTGCCCGTGC	-	Bsuc_PL10
9	TTCGAACTAGTTTGGACCATTCAACGAAATTATTTCGAGGTATCT	-	P$_{ldhA}$
10	CCTCGAAATAATTTCGTTGAATGGTCCAAACTAGTTCGAA + 4	-	Bsuc_PL10 / GFP
11	GCGGTGGCGGCCGCTCTAGACACCGAGTTCGAGGGC	-	Bsuc_PL11
12	TTCGAACTAGTTTGGACCATGCCAATTGTTGCATTTTTGTTACATA	-	P$_{sodC}$
13	ACAAAAATGCAACAATTGGCATGGTCCAAACTAGTTCGAA + 4	-	Bsuc_PL11 / GFP
14	TTAAAGAGGAGAAATTAAGCATGGTCCAAACTAGTTCGAA	-	Bsuc_PL104
15	TCTACTGGGGATCCGGGCCCTTATTTGTAGAGCTCATCCAT	-	P$_{EM7*}$
16	45 + TCGAACTAGTTTGGACCATGCTTAATTTCTCCTCTTTAACC	-	Bsuc_PL104 / GFP
17	TGACGTCGGGCCCGGTACCACGCGTTATAAGCCTTTTAATCTACGCACCTTTTT	-	Bsuc_PL16
18	AAAGAATTATTTTGTTTTTTGCGTGAATTCCTCCTGATTATGATTGAGACGATAA	-	US_lacZ-DD0810
19	GTCTCAATCATAATCAGGAGGAATTCACGCAAAAACAAAATAATTCTTTACTTA	-	Bsuc_PL16
20	AGGAAAGCGGCCTATGGAGTCTAGATGTTAAATGCCAAATACCTTCATCATTTGC	-	DS_lacZ-DD0810
21	TGACGTCGGGCCCGGTACCACGCGTTAATGTTACGGCACCTACTTATACGGTA	-	Bsuc_PL17
22	CGCACTTTGAGTGCGATTACAATTTGAGTGTAACTCCTACAACTTAAAATATCTC	-	US_lacZ-DD0759
23	ATTTTAAGTTGTAGGAGTTACACTCAAATTGTAATCGCACTCAAAGTGCGGTA	-	Bsuc_PL17
24	AGGAAAGCGGCCTATGGAGTCTAGATGGGTTTCAATTTTGCCAACTCCCAC	-	DS_lacZ-DD0759
25	CCACCGCGGTGGCGGCCGCTCTAGATTAATTTGTTAACCTTAACACTATTTTTTG	-	Bsuc_PL18
26	CTTCAAATAACGATGGATAAACATAATTCCTCCTGATCCTTATCAAGGATTTTAATGTGGAA	810*	P$_{lacY}$
27	CACATTAAAATCCTTGATAAGGATCAGGAGGAATTATGTTTATCCATCGTTATTTTGAAGACCCT	810*	Bsuc_PL18 / DD0810
28	GTAAATCTACTGGGGATCCGGGCCCCTAACGAGCCGGGTTGCTCC	-	
29	CGGTGGCGGCCGCTCTAGAACTAGTTGCGGTCGGTTTTTGCCGAATTTTATAAT	-	Bsuc_PL18
30	GTAAATCTACTGGGGATCCGGGCCCTTATAAAATCTGCAATCTGAAGTCGCAATG	-	P$_{DD0759}$-DD0759
31	CGGTGGCGGCCGCTCTAGAACTAGTAATTTAGATATGTACCATTTAGTAATTAAA	-	Bsuc_PL25
32	GTAAATCTACTGGGGATCCGGGCCCTCAAGCAACCTGTACCGG	-	P$_{pflD}$panD$_{eco}$
33	22 + GTAAATCTACTGGGGATCCGGGCCCCTAAATGCTTCTCGACGTCA	-	Bsuc_PL26 / P$_{pflD}$panD$_{cgl}$
34	ACGGTTCATATAATTAGCCAATCTCATATGTTGTTGACAATTAATCATCGGCATA	-	Bsuc_PL47
35	AATCTTACTTCCGAGGATGGTGCGCAGCATGCTTAATTTCTCCTCTTTAACC	-	P$_{EM7*}$
36	AACCCCTAGGTTAAAGAGGAGAAATTAAGCATGCTGCGCACCATCCT	-	Bsuc_PL47
37	ATCATCGGAAGTTAGAGAGCATATGCTAAATGCTTCTCGACGTCA	-	panD$_{cgl}$
38	ACGGTTCATATAATTAGCCAATCTCATATGTTGTTGACAATTAATCATCGGCACA	-	Bsuc_PL80
39	ATTTTGCTGCCCAAAATGGTGCGTAACATGCTTAATTTCTCCTCTTTAACC	-	P$_{EM7*}$

* 810 = RBS$_{810}$, originates directly upstream of the *DD0810* gene

23

MATERIAL AND METHODS

Table 3.5. Oligonucleotides used as primers for genetic engineering of *B. succiniciproducens* and plasmid or strain validation (continued).

#	5'-Sequence-3'	Site	Plasmid and amplicon
40	ACCCCTAGGTTAAAGAGGAGAAATTAAGCATGTTACGCACCATTTTGGG	-	Bsuc_PL80
41	ATCATCGGAAGTTAGAGAGCATATGTTAAATGCTACGGCTGGTTA	-	panD$_{cgl}$$^+$
42	TCATATAATTAGCCAATCTCATATGAATTTAGATATGTACCATTTAGTAATTAAA	-	Bsuc_PL86
43	CCCAAAATGGTGCGTAACATTTTTAATACTTCCTTCTTTTCTAG	-	P$_{pflD}$
44	AAAAGAAGGAAGTATTAAAAATGTTACGCACCATTTTGGG + 32	-	Bsuc_PL86 panD$_{cgl}$$^+$
45	GCGGTGGCGGCCGCTCTAGATTGTTGACAATTAATCATCGGC	-	Bsuc_PL105
46	GTTTTTTGTTCCTTAACCATGCTTAATTTCTCCTCTTTAACC	-	P$_{EM7*}$
47	TTAAAGAGGAGAAATTAAGCATGGTTAAGGAACAAAAAACCG	-	Bsuc_PL105
48	TCTACTGGGGATCCGGGCCCTCAAGATGCCAAAATCTTAGAA	-	panP$_{vna}$
49	CGGTGGCGGCCGCTCTAGA**ACTAGT**AATTTAGATATGTACCATTTAGTAATTAAA	SpeI	Bsuc_PL27 P$_{pflD}$bapta$^+$$_{ppu}$-
50	GTAAATCTACTGGGGATCC**GGGCCC**TCATCACTACTATTATTATTATTGAC	ApaI	P$_{pflD}$ydfG$^+$$_{eco}$
51	CATATGCTCTCTAACTTCCG	-	Bsuc_PL98
52	TTAAATGCTACGGCTGGTTA	-	Bsuc_PL80
53	**25 +** CCGGTTTCCGGCATATTCATGCTTAATTTCTCCTCTTTCTAAATGCTTCTCGAC GTCA	RBS$_{EM7*}$	Bsuc_PL52 P$_{EM7*}$-panD$_{cgl}$
54	TGACGTCGAGAAGCATTTAGAAAGAGGAGAAATTAAGCATGAATATGCCGGA AACCGG	RBS$_{EM7*}$	Bsuc_PL52 RBS$_{EM7*}$-
55	CCGGTCACCAACACAATCATGCTTAATTTCTCCTCTTTTTAATCAATCAAGTTT AAGGTTTCAC	RBS$_{EM7*}$	bapta$_{ppu}$$^+$
56	GTGAAACCTTAAACTTGATTGATTAAAAAGAGGAGAAATTAAGCATGATTGTGT TGGTGACCGG + 41	RBS$_{EM7*}$	Bsuc_PL52 RBS$_{EM7*}$- ydfG$_{cgl}$$^+$
57	TAACCAGCCGTAGCATTTAAAAAGAGGAGAAATTAAGCATGAATATG	-	Bsuc_PL98 RBS$_{EM7*}$-
58	CGGAAGTTAGAGAGCATATGTTATTGACGATGCACATTTAAAC	-	bapta$_{ppu}$$^+$- RBS$_{EM7*}$- ydfG$_{eco}$$^+$
59	TTTCAGACTGGTTCAGGATGAGCTCTGCGGTCGGTTTTTGCCGAA	-	Bsuc_PL87 200 bp US-
60	TATCAACAGGAGTCCAAGCGAGCTCTTATAAAATCTGCAATCTGAAGTCGC	-	lacZ-DD0759- lacZ-DD0759
61	TTTCAGACTGGTTCAGGATGAGCTCTTAATTTGTTAACCTTAACACTATT	-	Bsuc_PL88 200 bp US-
62	TATCAACAGGAGTCCAAGCGAGCTCCTAACGAGCCGGGTTGCT	-	lacY-DD0811- RBS$_{DD0810}$- lacZ-DD0810
63	AGAGGCCTGACGTCGGGCCCAAGTTCTATGCTAAATCCAATTTAA	-	Bsuc_PL94 Bsuc_PL95
64	ATCGTAATTATTGGGGACCCGCAACACTAGAAAAATCTAAAAATT	-	US_DD0789- sucrose PTS
65	TTAGATTTTTCTAGTGTTGCGGGTCCCCAATAATTACGAT	-	Bsuc_PL94
66	TTTTTGACTGATTTTTTAAATTAGAAAAATTCATCCAGCATC	-	Bsuc_PL95 P$_{neo}$neo
67	TGCTGGATGAATTTTTCTAATTTAAAAAATCAGTCAAAAAGACC	-	Bsuc_PL94 Bsuc_PL95
68	TGACGCGTGGTACCGGGCCCCCAAAAGTAAATGTTAAAAATATGT	-	DS_DD0789- sucrose PTS
69	CCTTTAACTCTTCGCCATCC	-	pJFF224 screening primer
70	CCGCTAAGCGATAGACTGTA	-	

24

Table 3.5. Oligonucleotides used as primers for genetic engineering of *B. succiniciproducens* and plasmid or strain validation (continued 2).

#	5'-Sequence-3'	Site	Plasmid and amplicon
71	GTGAACGGCAGGTATATGTG	-	Bsuc_PL94
72	TGCCGAAAATAAAGTCACGG	-	Bsuc_PL95 screening primer
73	GACCGTACATAAAAGTGCGG	-	*B. succiniciproducens* genome
74	TTTGCGTTAAAAGTGCGGTC	-	ΔDD0789-trehalose PTS::P*neoneo* 5'-screening primer
75	CCAGAGTATTTTTGCTCTGG	-	*B. succiniciproducens* genome
76	GCCGATATCGAACTGGATTA	-	ΔDD0789-trehalose PTS::P*neoneo* 3'-screening primer

3.4.2 Amplification, ligation and assembly of nucleic acids

For plasmid construction and strain validation, the amplification of targeted DNA molecules was conducted by PCR (Mullis et al., 1986), using a Tgradient Thermocycler (Analytik Jena AG, Jena, Germany). For insert construction, a Phusion HighFidelity Polymerase master mix (Thermo Fisher Scientific, Waltham, MA, USA) was used. Strain validation was conducted using a Phire Hot Start II PCR master mix (Thermo Fisher Scientific, Waltham, MA, USA). DNA elution from columns was conducted using sterile demineralized water, pre-warmed to 65 °C. The strategy of insert amplification and cloning by Gibson's Assembly (Gibson et al., 2009) for plasmid construction is depicted in **Figure 3.1**.

DNA amplification was conducted using a standard temperature profile. The initial denaturation step (3 min at 98 °C) was followed by 30 cycles of 0.5 min for denaturation at 98 °C, 0.5 min for annealing at the specified annealing temperature of the primer pair, determined by Wallace's rule (**Equation 1**) and a subsequent elongation step at 72 °C with an adjusted duration. The duration of the elongation step was based on the elongation activity of the polymerase (30 seconds for 1000 bp, Phusion and 15 seconds for 1000 bp, Phire) and the length of the target DNA. After a final elongation step for 4 min at 72 °C, the thermocycler stored the PCR mixtures at 8 °C.

$$T = 2 \cdot (A + T) + 4 \cdot (G + C) \qquad (1)$$

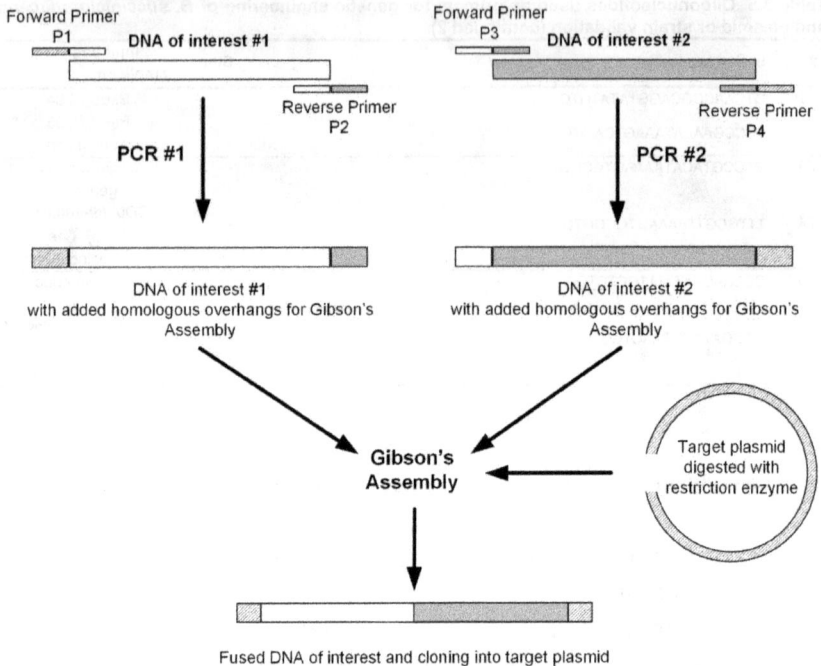

Figure 3.1. Strategy for nucleic acid amplification and subsequent cloning by Gibson's Assembly (Gibson et al., 2009). Target DNA is amplified by PCR using site-specific primers containing homologous regions of the parts to be fused. Therefore, PCR adds about 15-20 base pairs to the specific amplicon at each assembly region. After purification, the target DNA's are mixed with the appropriate and digested target plasmid. Finally, fusion of DNA of interest and cloning into plasmid is performed in one step by using Gibson's Assembly. The method was used to assemble up to three DNA parts (e.g. promoters in front of genes, or ribosomal binding sites in front of genes etc.).

DNA amplification for cloning efforts was carried out in 50 µL volume. For strain validation, amplification of DNA was conducted in a 15 µL volume. Primers were added to a final concentration of 200 nM. As a template, one µL of purified genomic DNA or plasmid DNA was used in cloning dependent reactions. Strain validations were performed by using at least one µL as template of a cell suspension of 20 µL, containing a single colony. Amplification reactions without addition of template DNA were used as negative controls. Positive controls were conducted with appropriate template DNA, if available. By addition of 5 % DMSO, DNA amplification was improved.

The Gibson's Assembly master mix was prepared according to literature and frozen in 15 µL aliquots at -20 °C (Gibson et al., 2009). After thawing an aliquot on ice, an appropriate vector-insert mixture (1:3 and 1:5, ad 5 µL with sterile demineralized water) was added. The reaction mix was incubated for 1 h at 50 °C and subsequently 5 µL were transformed into E. coli TOP10.

Ligation reactions were carried out with two different vector-insert ratios (1:3 and 1:5), using the RapidDNA ligation Kit (Roche Applied Science, Mannheim, Germany). The reaction mixtures were incubated for 30 min at room temperature. Subsequently, an aliquot of 5 µL was used for transformation in E. coli TOP10 by heat shock.

3.4.3 Gel electrophoresis

Amplification products from PCR or enzymatic restriction digestion assays were analyzed electrophoretically by separation in an 1 % agarose gel. In short, 1x TAE buffer (**Table 3.6**) was used for electrophoresis at 120 V for about 45 min (Easycast™ B1A or D2 gel system, Thermo Scientific, Marietta, OH, USA with PowerPac™ 300 BioRad Laboratories, Hercules, CA, USA). For the differentiation of band sizes, a 1 kb DNA ladder (O'GeneRuler™ 1 kb DNA ladder ready-to-use, Fermentas, St. Leon-Roth, Germany) was used. The samples were mixed in a 1:10 ratio with OrangeG (**Table 3.6**) loading dye prior to gel loading. After DNA separation, the gels were stained in an ethidium bromide dye bath (0.5 µg mL^{-1} ethidium bromide). The detection of DNA was conducted under UV light (Universell Hood II T2A, BioRad Laboratories, Hercules, CA, USA).

Table 3.6. Buffer composition used for gel electrophoresis.

Buffer	Composition
10x Orange G	20 g Sucrose 100 mg OrangeG ad 50 mL H$_2$O
50x TAE	242 g Tris-base 57.1 mL glacial acetate 37.2 g Na$_2$EDTA·H$_2$O pH 8 ad 1000 mL H$_2$O

3.4.4 Enzymatic digestion

For the validation of cloning experiments, the preparation of suitable vectors for Gibson's Assembly or ligation based cloning, plasmid DNA or amplified target DNA was digested using selected restriction enzymes (FastDigest series, Thermo Fisher Scientific, Waltham, MA, USA), respectively. The digestion of plasmid DNA (10 µg) or linear DNA (4 µg) for cloning was conducted in a total volume of 20 µL. For analytical digestions, 500 ng plasmid DNA was used. Digestion of plasmid DNA was performed at 37 °C overnight. Linear DNA or analytical digests were incubated at 37 °C for 1.5 h. Subsequently, linearized vectors for ligation based cloning were treated by alkaline phosphatase (Shrimp alkaline phosphatase (SAP), Roche Applied Science, Mannheim, Germany). The reaction mixture was incubated 40 min at room temperature to eliminate the phosphate residue, which avoided cloning dependent re-ligation of the vector.

3.4.5 Transformation

The preparation of heat shock competent E. coli TOP10 cells was based on literature (Inoue et al., 1990). For heat shock transformation, an aliquot (50 µL) of competent cells was thawed on ice. Subsequently, 1 µL plasmid DNA or 5 µL ligation- or Gibson's Assembly dependent cloning reaction was added. The mixture was stored for 30 min on ice and was subsequently heat-shocked at 45 °C for 45 seconds. Afterwards, the mixture was stored on ice for another 5 min. Then, 950 µL of sterile LB medium was added for the regeneration (37 °C, 900 rpm, 1 h) of the cells (Thermomixer comfort, Eppendorf, Hamburg, Germany). Finally, the cells were plated on LB agar plates, containing 10 µg mL^{-1} chloramphenicol and were incubated at 37 °C overnight. Obtained colonies were validated, using PCR or restriction digestion assays, as specified before.

For each electroporation of plasmid DNA, competent cells of B. succiniciproducens were freshly obtained by aerobic cultivation in baffled shake flasks. A pre-grown overnight BHI culture (10 mL, 37 °C, 230 rpm) inoculated from a glycerol stock, was used to inoculate the main culture (50 mL, 37 °C, 230 rpm) to an initial OD$_{600}$ of 0.05. During cultivation OD$_{600}$ was measured and the cells were harvested at a final OD$_{600}$ of 0.3 by centrifugation (5000 x g, 10 min, 4 °C). Subsequently, the cells were washed with 50 mL ice-cold 10 % glycerol and harvested equally. The cell pellet was suspended in 1 mL ice-cold 10 % glycerol. Aliquots of 100 µL cell suspension were then mixed with plasmid DNA (2 µg). The mixture was electroporated with a MicroPulser electroporator (BioRad Laboratories, Hercules, CA, USA) at 2 kV, 400 Ω and 25 µF. After the pulse, pre-warmed BHI was added to a final volume of 1 mL and the cells were regenerated for 1.5 h (37 °C, 550 rpm, Thermomixer comfort, Eppendorf, Hamburg, Germany). Subsequently, the cells were plated on buffered BHI agar plates, containing 5 µg mL^{-1} chloramphenicol and incubated for up to 48 h at 37 °C.

3.4.6 Strain validation

Colonies, obtained from the transformation were validated by PCR, regarding the presence of the episomal plasmid (pJFF224-XN based transformation), using the primer pair 69 and 70 (**Table 3.5**). This primer pair was designed for amplification of the multiple cloning site region of pJFF224-XN to detect cloning based assembly events or the resulting specific plasmid fingerprints in transformed strains.

First recombination events (pClik^{CM} based transformation) were validated with specific primer pairs (**Table 3.5, Figure 3.2**). Subsequently, second recombination events (pClik^{CM} based transformation) in positive clones from the first recombination, were initiated by cultivation in BHI medium (25 mL, 37 °C, 230 rpm, 48 h) without selection pressure. Aliquots of the cultures were plated in dilutions from 10^{-3} to 10^{-6} on buffered BHI agar plates. After incubation overnight at 37 °C, clones were selected and validated by PCR, using specific primer pairs (**Table 3.5**).

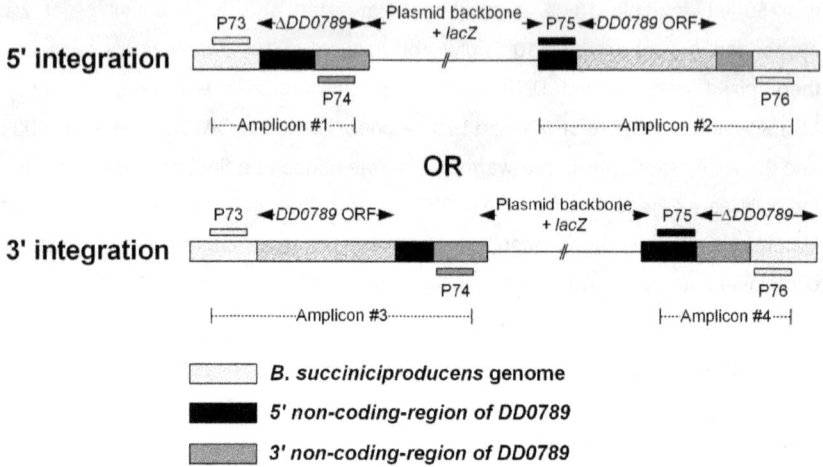

Figure 3.2. Strain validation of first recombination events in *B. succiniciproducens* DD3ΔΔ*lacZ*. The deletion plasmid of the target gene *DD0789* can enter the *B. succiniciproducens* genome via homologous recombination in 5'- or 3'-integration direction. The primer pairs 73 + 74 and 75 + 76 enable a direct analysis of integration direction by PCR. As well, the *lacZ* genes on Bsuc_PL94 and Bsuc_PL95 enable a direct visible screening on buffered BHI agar plates with X-gal. The latter turns first recombination colonies blue. Second recombination events can be validated by using the mentioned primer pairs. The parent strain *B. succiniciproducens* DD3ΔΔ*lacZ* forms white colonies on buffered BHI with X-gal, when plasmid loss occurred, and consequently plasmid based *lacZ* activity is eliminated.

3.4.7 Strain preservation

Obtained strains during strain construction were inoculated on appropriate agar plates. After incubation of about 12 – 18 h at 37 °C, cells were harvested and suspended in 1.2 mL of a buffer solution containing per Liter: 3.75 g (*N*-morpholino)propanesulfonic acid (MOPS), 0.25 g Mg(OH)$_2$, 2.30 g 2,2-*Bis*(hydroxymethyl)-2,2',2"nitrilotriethanol (Bis-Tris) and 0.72 g NaHCO$_3$. After complete resuspension of the cells, 0.4 mL of 80 % glycerol was added and the glycerol stock was frozen and stored at -80 °C.

3.5 Cultivation and strain characterization

3.5.1 Aerobic cultivation in shake flasks

The first pre-culture was inoculated from a glycerol stock and incubated overnight at 37 °C on an orbital shaker (230 rpm, 5 cm shaking diameter, Infors Multitron, Bottmingen, Switzerland) in 100 mL baffled shake-flasks, filled with 10 mL medium. Subsequently, cells were harvested (5 min, 5000x g, 25 °C), washed once with medium and then used to inoculate the second pre-culture to an initial cell concentration (OD_{600}) of 0.1, which was incubated for 3 h as described above, followed again by harvesting. Main cultures were then inoculated to an initial cell concentration (OD_{600}) of 0.2 and were grown as triplicates in 500 mL baffled shake flasks, filled with 50 mL medium (**Table 3.3**), as given above.

Cultivation for promoter screening (BHI medium + 10 g L^{-1} glucose), media development and kanamycin resistance screening was conducted in a miniaturized and parallelized bioreactor system with online sensing of fluorescence (excitation 460 nm, emission 520 nm), cell concentration as optical density (OD_{620}) at 620 nm, dissolved oxygen level and pH of the culture broth (m2p-labs, Hauppauge, NY, USA). Here, the incubation was conducted at 37 °C and 1000 rpm. For the determination of promoter strength, the fluorescence signal was plotted against the cell concentration. The slope derived from the correlation was assigned to the specific promoter activity under the given conditions (Alper et al., 2005). *B. succiniciproducens* DD3 + pJFF224, harboring the empty plasmid, was used as negative control to correct for background fluorescence. All experiments were conducted in triplicates.

3.5.2 Anaerobic cultivation in serum bottles

Growth experiments were conducted in a glucose-based minimal-medium with $MgCO_3$ as buffer system (**Table 3.4**). Routine cultivations were conducted in 30 mL serum bottles, filled with 10 mL medium. A CO_2 atmosphere with 0.8 bar overpressure was applied and the bottles were sealed with gas-tight butyl rubber stoppers (Becker et al., 2013).

The first pre-culture was seeded with an inoculation loop from an agar plate culture grown in a CO_2 enriched atmosphere at 37 °C (Anaerocult® C mini, Merck Millipore, Darmstadt, Germany) and was then incubated overnight at 37 °C on an orbital shaker

(230 rpm, 5 cm shaking diameter, Infors Multitron, Bottmingen, Switzerland). Subsequently, cells from exponential growth phase were harvested (5 min, 5000 x g, 25 °C), washed once with medium and were then used to inoculate the main culture to an initial cell concentration (OD_{600}) of 0.5, grown in triplicates.

For defined alanine production experiments, exponentially growing cells were switched to an atmosphere of either CO_2 or N_2 at 0.8 bar overpressure. Therefore, 10 mL of an aerobic main culture at a cell dry mass of about 0.8 g L^{-1} was transferred in serum bottles equipped with gas-tight butyl rubber stoppers and the atmosphere switch was applied. Experiments were conducted in triplicates.

3.5.3 Cultivation in lab scale bioreactors

Bioreactor cultivations were carried out in batch and in fed-batch mode, respectively, using lab scale bioreactors (DasGIP, Eppendorf AG, Hamburg, Germany). Batch processes for L-alanine production were conducted at 37 °C in parallelized 250 mL reactors, filled with 40 mL medium (**Table 3.3**). The process was maintained at pH 7.0 by automatic addition of 25 % NH_4OH and was operated either under anaerobic conditions (0.18 vvm N_2) or under microaerobic conditions (without aeration) (Yamamoto et al., 2012). The stirring rate was set to 400 min^{-1} throughout the process. After 2 hours, a pulse of $(NH_4)_2SO_4$ was added, supplying a concentration of 10 g L^{-1} from a sterilized stock solution (500 g L^{-1}, pH 7.2).

The fed-batch process for L-alanine production was conducted using 1 L bioreactors, filled initially with 300 mL batch medium (**Table 3.3**) with differing concentrations of the carbon source, which was 15 g or 30 g xylose as given below. The process was again operated at 37 °C and pH 7.0. Different culture regimes were chosen: (i) initial aerobic phase (1.8 vvm pressurized air) and subsequent anaerobic phase (1.8 vvm N_2), and (ii) completely anaerobic process (1.8 vvm N_2). After the initially added xylose was depleted, the feed phase was started. The feed was added pulse-wise on basis of external xylose measurement, to keep the substrate level between 5 and 15 g L^{-1}. The feed solution contained per liter: 450 g xylose, 200 g $(NH_4)_2SO_4$, 4 mL Na_2CO_3 stock solution (250 g L^{-1}), 5 g yeast extract (Becton Dickinson), 5 g BHI (Becton Dickinson), 5 mL glycine-betaine stock solution (58.6 g L^{-1}), 3 g K_2HPO_4, 5 mL 200x trace element stock solution (10 g L^{-1} $FeSO_4 \cdot 7H_2O$, 2.0 g L^{-1} $CaCl_2 \cdot 2H_2O$, 0.4 g L^{-1} $MnSO_4 \cdot H_2O$, 2.2 g L^{-1} $ZnSO_4 \cdot 7H_2O$, 1.0 g L^{-1} $CuSO_4 \cdot 5H_2O$, 0.02 g L^{-1} $Na_2B_4O_7 \cdot 10H_2O$,

0.1 g L^{-1} (NH$_4$)$_6$Mo$_7$O$_{24}$·4H$_2$O) and 10 mL of a 100x vitamin stock solution (10 g L^{-1} Ca-pantothenate, 0.5 g L^{-1} biotin, 0.05 g L^{-1} cyanocobalamin, 3 g L^{-1} nicotinamide, 1 g L^{-1} pyridoxal·HCl, 0.6 g L^{-1} riboflavin and 3 g L^{-1} thiamin·HCl) (Becker et al., 2013; Young Lee, 1996). All processes were conducted in duplicates.

3.6 Analytical methods

3.6.1 Cell and biomass concentration

The cell concentration was measured as optical density (OD$_{600}$) at 600 nm in duplicates (1600 PC, VWR, Darmstadt, Germany). The cell dry mass (CDM) was inferred from the optical density as previously described (Becker et al., 2013). An OD$_{600}$-CDM correlation factor of 0.331 g$_{CDM}$ OD$_{600}$$^{-1}$ was used.

3.6.2 Substrates and products

Glucose, fructose, sucrose, xylose, glycerol, pyruvate, lactate, acetate, 3-hydroxypropionate, and succinate were quantified by HPLC in 1:5 diluted samples (Agilent 1260 Infinity Series, Agilent Technologies, Waldbronn, Germany) on an HPX-87H (Bio-Rad, Hercules, CA, USA) at 55 °C with 0.5 mM H$_2$SO$_4$ at 0.7 mL min^{-1} as mobile phase and refraction index detection (Agilent 1260, RID G1362A, Agilent Technologies) with external standards. Amino acids were quantified by HPLC using 1:10 diluted samples with α-aminobutyric acid as internal standard (Agilent 1200 Series, Agilent Technologies), involving pre-column derivatization with o-phthalaldehyde, separation on a Gemini C18 column (Phenomenex, Aschaffenburg, Germany) by gradient elution (A: 4.8 g L^{-1} NaH$_2$PO$_4$, 0.5 g L^{-1} NaN$_3$, B: 45 % acetonitrile, 45 % methanol, 10 % deionized water, gradient: 0 - 27.5 minutes at 100 % A, 27.5 - 28 minutes at 72.5 % A and 27.5 % B, 28 - 32 minutes at 100 % B, 32 - 37 minutes at 100 % A) at a flow rate of 1 mL min^{-1} and fluorescence detection (Krömer et al., 2005).

3.6.3 GC-MS labeling analysis

The analysis and identification of secreted products except acetate was conducted by GC/MS (5977A MSD, 7890B GC, HP-5MS capillary column, 30 m x 250 µm, Agilent Technologies, Waldbronn, Germany). In short, 50 µL of a culture supernatant was dried under a nitrogen stream (Wittmann et al., 2002). The obtained residue was re-dissolved in 50 µL dimethyl formamide (0.1 % pyridine), then mixed with 50 µL N-methyl-N-*t*-butyl-dimethylsilyl-trifluoroacetamide (MBDSTFA) (Macherey-Nagel, Düren, Germany) and converted into the *t*-butyl-dimethylsilyl (TBMDS) derivatives for 30 minutes at 80 °C.

The instrument was operated at a carrier gas flow of 1.7 mL min^{-1} and temperatures of 250 °C (inlet), 230 °C (interface), and 150 °C (quadrupole). The temperature gradient for separation was 120 °C for 2 minutes, a ramp of 8 °C min^{-1} up to 200 °C, and then 10 °C min^{-1} up to 325 °C. GC-MS measurement was first conducted in scan mode (*m/z* 50 – 750). The quantitative analysis of the ^{13}C labeling pattern of TBDMS-amino acids glycine (246 *m/z*), valine (288 *m/z*), leucine (302 *m/z*), isoleucine (302 *m/z*), serine (390 *m/z*), threonine (404 *m/z*), phenylalanine (336 *m/z*), aspartate (418 *m/z*), lysine (431 *m/z*) and tyrosine (466 *m/z*) was carried out in selected ion monitoring (SIM) mode. The analyzed ion cluster at *m/z* 260 – 264 represents a fragment ion, which contains the entire carbon skeleton and the amino group of alanine (Wittmann, 2007) and β-alanine as well as the entire carbon skeleton of 3-HP and lactate. Succinate was also considered (289 *m/z*). Measurements concerning acetate were derivatized with n-pentanol and measured according to (Adler et al., 2013).

3.6.4 Enzyme activities

Cells were disrupted (Precellys, VWR, Erlangen, Germany) using Lysing matrix B tubes (MP biomedicals, Eschwege, Germany) in 100 mM Tris/HCl (pH 7.8, 1 mM dithiothreitol). Alanine dehydrogenase was assayed after adding 50 µL cell extract to 950 µL of a reaction mixture, containing 100 mM Tris/HCl (pH 9.0), 0.25 mM NADH, 5 mM $(NH_4)_2SO_4$, and 10 mM pyruvate (Germano and Anderson, 1968).

Aspartate 1-decarboxylase (PanD, PanP) activity was detected via β-alanine formation in HPLC measurements. For measurement of PanD, 100 µL cell extract were added to 1.9 mL of a 100 mM potassium phosphate buffer (pH 6.8) containing 1.2 mM L-aspartate. To measure PanP, a buffer variation was used (100 mM potassium phosphate buffer (pH 7.5), 10 mM L-aspartate, 5 mM $MgSO_4$ and 0.75 mM pyridoxal 5-phosphate) (Pan et al., 2017). The mixture was incubated at 30 °C and 500 rpm (Thermomixer comfort, Eppendorf, Hamburg, Germany) and 100 µL samples were withdrawn in specific intervals up to 5 h. Subsequently the samples were inactivated at 100 °C for 5 min (Thermomixer comfort, Eppendorf, Hamburg, Germany) and diluted 1:10 with α-aminobutyric acid as an internal standard and measured with HPLC as described above.

Glucose 6-phosphate (G6P) dehydrogenase activity was determined after adding 50 µL cell extract to 950 µL of a reaction mixture containing 100 mM Tris/HCl (pH 7.8), 10 mM $MgCl_2$, 1 mM $NADP^+$, 5 mM glucose 6-phosphate (Becker et al., 2013).

Negative controls for each assay were conducted without cell extract or substrate, respectively. The total protein concentration was determined using the bicinchoninic acid assay (Smith et al., 1985). One unit of enzyme activity was defined as the amount of enzyme, converting 1 µmol of NAD^+ (alanine dehydrogenase) or $NADP^+$ (G6P dehydrogenase), which was quantified via the absorption change at 340 nm. The latter was also defined for β-alanine formation activity. All assays were conducted in triplicates at 30 °C.

4   RESULTS AND DISCUSSION

4.1   Growth physiology of *Basfia succiniciproducens* DD3 under aerobic and anaerobic conditions

Initial studies investigated the basic properties and production characteristics of *B. succiniciproducens*. These studies were conducted with the strain *B. succiniciproducens* DD3, lacking the *ldhA* and the *pflD* gene (Becker et al., 2013). The elimination of the by-products lactate and formate, achieved by the double deletion, previously led to high succinate production. Here, it appeared also promising towards overproduction of carbon-three chemicals.

To get an insight into the growth physiology, anaerobic cultivation in glucose minimal medium was performed (**Figure 4.1**). The strain grew from early on and mainly produced within 48 h, 33.0 ± 0.9 g L^{-1} succinate from 50 g L^{-1} glucose. Acetate $(2.0 \pm 0.0$ g L^{-1}, $Y_{acetate/glucose} = 0.05 \pm 0.00$ $g_{acetate}$ $g_{glucose}^{-1})$, pyruvate $(2.6 \pm 0.0$ g L^{-1}, $Y_{pyruvate/glucose} = 0.07 \pm 0.00$ $g_{pyruvate}$ $g_{glucose}^{-1})$ and traces of formate, lactate and ethanol were found as by-products. In the exponential growth phase a μ_{max} of 0.07 ± 0.01 h^{-1} was derived. The biomass yield $Y_{X/S}$ was low $(0.07 \pm 0.01$ g_{CDM} $g_{glucose}^{-1})$, indicating only partial conversion of glucose into biomass. The specific glucose consumption rate (q_S) was 0.99 ± 0.04 $g_{glucose}$ g_{CDM}^{-1} h^{-1}. The generation time was determined to be 10.3 ± 1.4 h^{-1}. The succinate-substrate yield $(0.66 \pm 0.01$ $g_{succinate}$ $g_{glucose}^{-1})$ was highly similar to previous findings (Becker et al., 2013).

The deletion of competing fermentative pathways is a common strategy for enhancing succinate production (Lee et al., 2006; Litsanov et al., 2012; Zhu et al., 2014). The detected pyruvate indicated an intracellular excess of pyruvate and an overflow at the pyruvate node (Becker et al., 2013). This suggested a good start point into metabolic engineering of *B. succiniciproducens* for pyruvate-derived products (Becker et al., 2015).

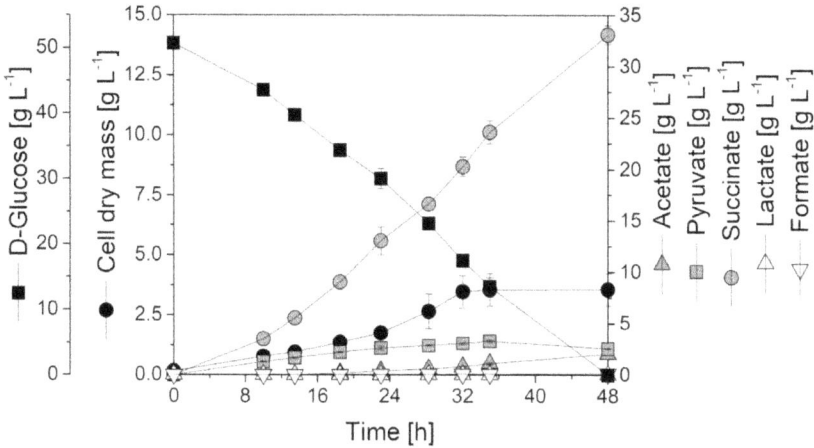

Figure 4.1. Anaerobic cultivation profile of *B. succiniciproducens* DD3 in glucose minimal medium. The data represent three independent replicates with means and deviation.

In comparison, the aerobic cultivation of *B. succiniciproducens* DD3 in complex growth medium revealed a rapid increase in cell concentration, associated with a μ_{max} of 0.81 ± 0.02 h^{-1} (**Figure 4.2**). This growth rate corresponded to a generation time of 52 ± 1 min. The biomass yield was 0.23 ± 0.02 g_{CDM} $g_{glucose}^{-1}$. The cells exhibited a rapid glucose consumption corresponding to a glucose consumption rate q_s of 3.5 ± 0.2 $g_{glucose}$ g_{CDM}^{-1} h^{-1}. In contrast to the anaerobic cultivation, acetate $(6.4 \pm 0.1$ g $L^{-1})$ was the dominating product instead of succinate $(2.3 \pm 0.5$ g $L^{-1})$. Only traces of other by-products were observed.

It is assumed, that the double deletion of the *ldhA* and *pflD* gene in *B. succiniciproducens* DD3 leads to the strong acetate production. In contrast, aerobic cultivation of wild type *Mannheimia succiniciproducens*, containing functional copies of *ldhA* and *pflD*, showed a strong lactate production (Lee et al., 2002).

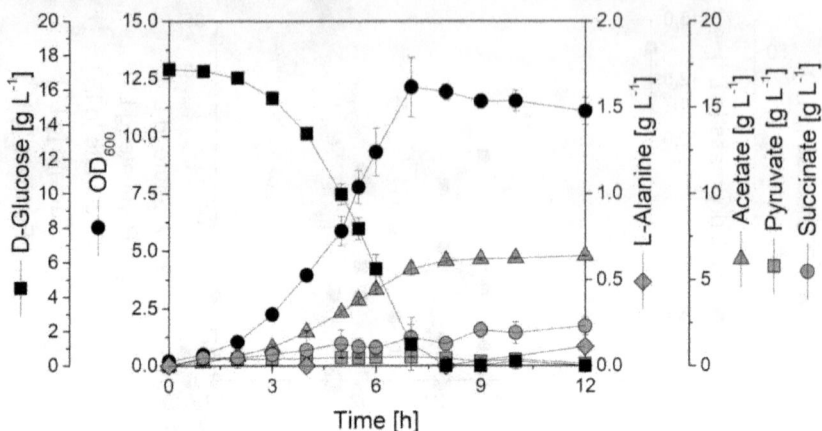

Figure 4.2. Aerobic growth physiology of *B. succiniciproducens* DD3 in shake flask. Measurement of organic acids, sugars and amino acids was conducted using HPLC. The data represent three independent replicates with means and deviation.

The pronounced production of acetate indicated an increased availability of carbon at the pyruvate pool. This appeared promising to establish new pathways for other pyruvate-derived products, using *B. succiniciproducens*. The observed product shift to acetate is also prominent in aerobically growing *E. coli* under excess glucose (Luli and Strohl, 1990). It is thought to be a limitation in respiratory capacity (Andersen and von Meyenburg, 1980; Szenk et al., 2017) enabling the cell to gain additional ATP, using substrate level phosphorylation involving the *pta-ackA* pathway.

4.2 Development of genetic tools for *Basfia succiniciproducens*

4.2.1 Development of a blue-white screening system for genomic engineering

Different experiments aimed to develop a method for more convenient genome engineering of *B. succiniciproducens* (Becker et al., 2013; Lange et al., 2017). This appeared reasonable, because genomic modification in this microbe is not yet well established. So far, genomic modification is exclusively done via homologous recombination, using homologous non-coding genomic regions located on the integrative vector pClik^{CM} (Becker et al., 2013). The lack of an efficient selection marker makes engineering efforts time-consuming and elaborative. To speed up existing protocols, the development of a suitable screening system for genomic modification of *B. succiniciproducens* was targeted in the present study.

Since blue white screening has been established for cloning efforts (Vieira and Messing, 1982), many applications and variations of this technique emerged (Geng et al., 2016; Speltz and Regan, 2013). Basically, the technique utilizes the expression of a β-galactosidase (LacZ), which turns clone colonies blue, upon the cleavage of a D-lactose analog, i.e. 5-bromo-4-chloro-3-indolyl-β-D-galactopyranoside, yielding galactose and 5-bromo-4-chloro-3-hydroxyindole (Kiernan, 2007). The latter dimerizes to 5,5'-dibromo-4,4'-dichloro-indigo, an insoluble blue stain. After cloning of target DNA into the artificial open reading frame of the β-galactosidase gene (*lacZ*) on the cloning vector, β-galactosidase expression and activity diminishes (Sambrook, 2001). This enables a convenient and efficient identification of recombinant clones. This system should now be applied to *B. succiniciproducens* for genomic engineering.

One example for blue-white selection was conducted within the rumen bacterium *A. succinogenes* in 2014 (Joshi et al., 2014) which is also a member of *Pasteurellaceae* family. Here, deletion of the native β-galactosidase *lacZ* gene copy from the *A. succinogenes* genome revealed a possible blue-white selection for Δ*lacZ* recombinants. However, this was only restricted to construction of the Δ*pflB* Δ*lacZ* strain (Joshi et al., 2014) and not for general construction approaches.

4.2.2 *Basfia succiniciproducens* contains two β-galactosidase genes

The basis for blue white selection is a commonly known β-galactosidase gene *lacZ*, exclusively subcloned on common cloning vectors. Two candidate genes for native β-galactosidases were annotated in the genome of *B. succiniciproducens*. Like *B. succiniciproducens*, its relative *M. succiniciproducens* contains also two *lacZ* genes which seem to posess a critical role in lactose metabolism and further unknown functions (Lee et al., 2012). But blue-white screening technique is not described in literature for *M. succiniciproducens*.

The genes *DD0759* (*lacZ1*, 3042 bp) and *DD0810* (*lacZ2*, 3027 bp) were annotated as β-galactosidases when BLAST was performed on the DNA and protein level (**Table 4.1**). The two genes differed in similarity on the DNA (37 %) and on the protein level (44 %). It seemed that both genes were also paralogues (Lee et al., 2012). The corresponding proteins showed strong similarity when compared to the genes and proteins of the related bacterium *M. succiniciproducens* MBEL55E. The next similar genes were found in the family of *Pasteurellaceae* varying from 70 % on DNA level to 59 % on protein level (**Table 4.1**). This showed the narrow relation of *B. succiniciproducens* and *M. succiniciproducens* as indicated by the distinct differences between the gene and protein sequences of other *Pasteurellaceae* (**Table 4.1**).

Table 4.1. Overview of gene properties of two native *B. succiniciproducens lacZ* genes and BLAST similarities to related strains. The native *B. succiniciproducens lacZ* genes were compared to the three most related genes by KEGG BLAST on DNA and protein level.

Gene	Length (bp)	DNA similarity, gene, strain	Protein similarity, protein, strain
DD0759	3042	**99 %**, *MS0749*, *M. succiniciproducens* MBEL55E **70 %**, *PARA_19840*, *Haemophilus parainfluenzae* T3T1 **70 %**, *X874_17500*, *Mannheimia variegena* USDA-ARS-USMARC-1312	**99 %**, LacZ, *M. succiniciproducens* MBEL55E **64 %**, β-D-galactosidase, *Haemophilus parainfluenzae* T3T1 **60 %**, β-galactosidase, *Mannheimia variegena* USDA-ARS-USMARC-1312
DD0810	3027	**99 %**, *MS0806*, *M. succiniciproducens* MBEL55E **69 %**, *Asuc_1398*, *A. succinogenes* 130Z **69 %**, *K756_07455*, *Haemophilus parasuis* ZJ0906	**99 %**, LacZ, *M. succiniciproducens* MBEL55E **61 %**, glycoside hydrolase family 2 TIM barrel, *A. succinogenes* 130Z **59 %**, β-galactosidase, *Haemophilus parasuis* ZJ0906

The β-galactosidase was active *in vivo*. When *B. succiniciproducens* DD3 was streaked on agar supplemented with X-gal, β-galactosidase activity was observable indicated by the blue color (**Figure 4.3 A**). To establish a suitable blue-white screening system, the deletion of all endogenous *lacZ* genes was required (Barton, 2015). The single deletion of neither *DD0759* nor *DD0810* had an effect on the X-gal cleavage ability. Only the double deletion of both genes *DD0759* and *DD0810* yielded a strain, which had lost the X-gal cleavage ability (**Figure 4.3 B**). As a further proof-of-concept, this could be restored with complementation plasmids (Bsuc_PL18 and Bsuc_PL19), containing either the *DD0759* or the *DD0810* gene under the native promoter control, respectively (**Figure 4.3 C+D**) (Barton, 2015). This proved that both endogenic *lacZ* genes enabled X-gal cleavage, so the corresponding mutants exhibited β-galactosidase activity.

The blue-white screening strain, designated *B. succiniciproducens* DD3ΔΔ*lacZ*, was now used to establish a more convenient genomic modification method for *B. succiniciproducens*.

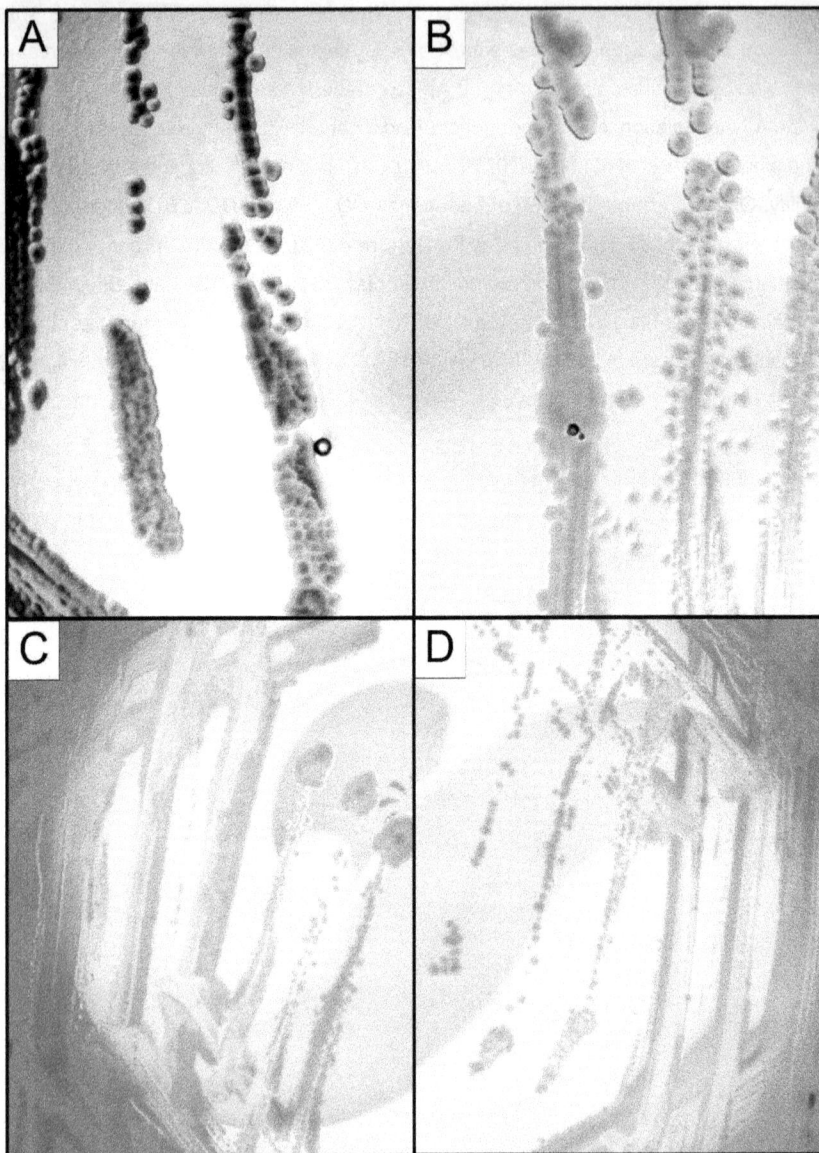

Figure 4.3. Comparison of *B. succiniciproducens* DD3 and DD3Δ*DD0759*Δ*DD0810*. The strains DD3 (**A**) and DD3Δ*DD0759*Δ*DD0810* lacking the *lacZ* genes *DD0759* and *DD0810* (**B**), were streaked on buffered BHI agar containing 80 µg mL^{-1} X-gal. The double *lacZ* knockout strain showed a lack of β-galactosidase activity (**B**). This property was restored, when gene function was complemented using the native *lacZ* genes, *DD0810* (**C**) or *DD0759* (**D**), on the episomal vector pJFF224-XN under native promoter control.

4.2.3 Modification of the integrative pClik^{CM} vector for blue-white screening

As shown, X-gal cleavage ability was restored by the episomal plasmids Bsuc_PL18 and Bsuc_PL19. In a next step, these findings were implemented into the integrative vector pClik^{CM}, a commonly used vector for genomic modification of *B. succiniciproducens* and other microorganisms (Becker et al., 2013; Becker et al., 2011; Lange et al., 2017). The idea was to provide one of the identified β-galactosidase genes on the pClik^{CM} backbone. In case of the occurrence of homologous recombination, cells which then contain a genomic copy of the modified vector should turn blue. If the vector was excised in a second recombination event the colonies should again turn white, consequently.

First, derivatives of pClik^{CM} containing one of the *B. succiniciproducens lacZ* genes on the vector backbone, each with its native promoter, were cloned into the multiple cloning site of the linearized (*SacI*) pClik^{CM} vector. This yielded the integrative plasmids Bsuc_PL87 and Bsuc_PL88, containing either *DD0759* or *DD0810*, respectively. Remarkably is, that positive clone colonies of the cloning host *E. coli* TOP10 were highlighted by the blue color on LB agar supplemented with X-gal (**Figure 4.4 A + B**). These clones contained the version of Bsuc_PL87 and Bsuc_PL88 episomally. This was emphasized in comparison with clones containing episomal pClik^{CM}, missing X-gal cleavage (**Figure 4.4 C**). Here, convenience of using blue-white screening is demonstrated, but validation was furthermore conducted by PCR.

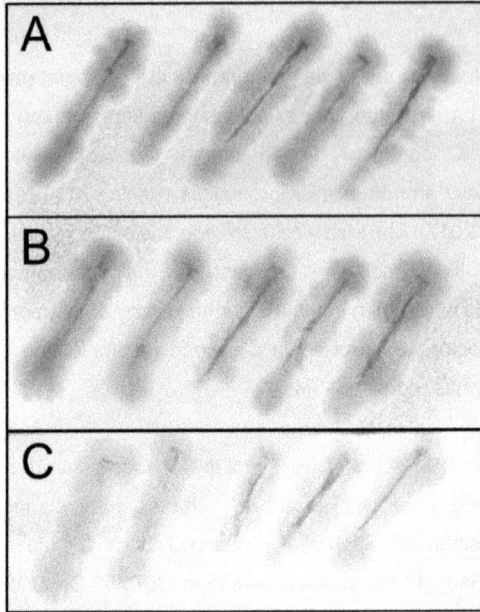

Figure 4.4. Clones of the intermediate host *E. coli* TOP10 containing the plasmids Bsuc_PL087 and Bsuc_PL088 episomally. The genes *DD0759-lacZ* and *DD0810-lacZ* with their native control elements (promoters) were cloned into the linearized (*SacI*) vector pClik^{CM} (**A + B**). Selection of positive clones was verified by blue-white screening on LB CM agar containing 80 μg mL^{-1} X-gal and comparison to clones containing the non-modified vector pClik^{CM} (**C**).

The modifications of the pClik^{CM} vector should now enable a blue-white screening for *B. succiniciproducens* (**Figure 4.5**). The strategy comprises the cloning of homologous regions of a deletion target gene (**Figure 4.5 A, Case 1.**) into the multiple cloning site (MCS) of Bsuc_PL87 or Bsuc_PL88. The modified vectors now indicated their genomic integration after a first recombination event by turning recombinant clone colonies blue, when incubated with X-gal. In addition, this should also enable the screening for homologous integration of DNA sequences of choice, e.g. genes or promoters (**Figure 4.5 A, Case 2.**). This reduces the effort to screen for false-positive clones after the first recombination (**Figure 4.5 B**). In the second recombination, the vector excision should again yield white clone colonies, indicating a modified mutant strain or the wild type strain (**Figure 4.5 C**). Only the obtained white clones are validated using PCR, which reduces the amount of screened colonies lacking the second recombination event. The developed strategy was now validated in a strain engineering approach.

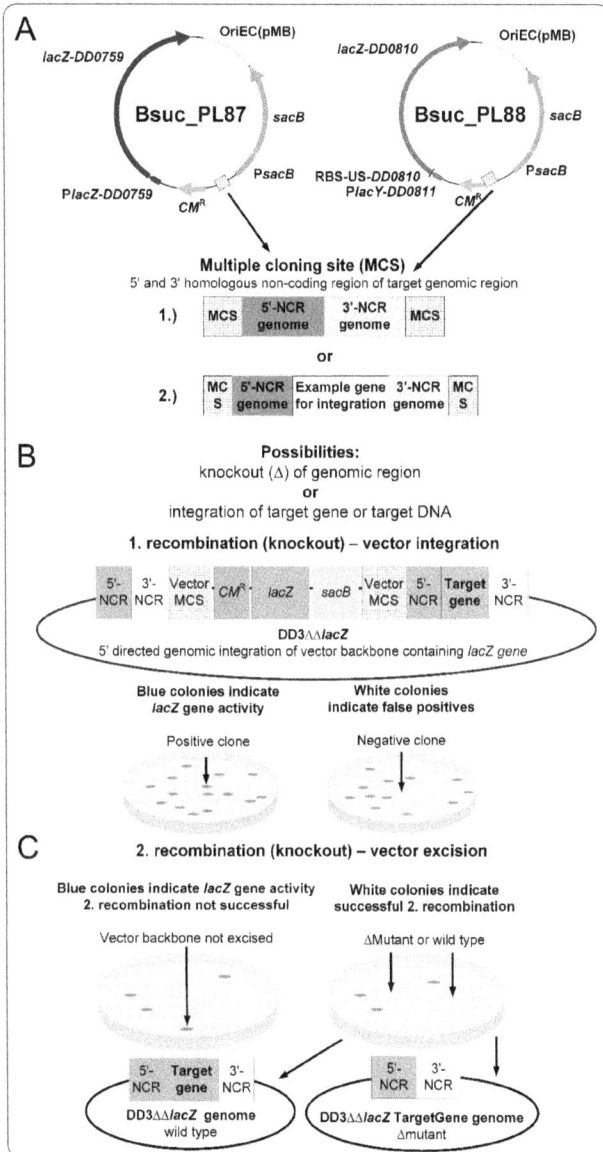

Figure 4.5. Theoretical background for blue-white screening using *B. succiniciproducens* DD3ΔΔ*lacZ*. To establish blue-white screening, the integrative vector pClik[CM] (Becker et al., 2013) was modified by cloning the *lacZ-DD0759* and *lacZ-DD0810* genes on the vector backbone under native promoter control, respectively. Furthermore, modification for heterologous recombination by using non-coding regions of target genes enable genomic modification (**A**). This is the basis for genomic modification of *B. succiniciproducens* DD3ΔΔ*lacZ*. The genomic integration of the vector is highlighted by turning clone colonies blue through *lacZ* gene activity after X-gal incubation (**B**). Modified strains (or wild type) should again yield white clone colonies after excision of the vector in 2. recombination (**C**).

4.2.4 Application of blue-white screening to gene deletion

The deletion of the target gene *DD0789* in *B. succiniciproducens* DD3ΔΔ*lacZ*, which is similar to the *M. succiniciproducens* sucrose PTS transporter *MS0784* (Lee et al., 2010), should demonstrate the potential of the blue-white screening strategy. The design included the replacement of *DD0789* by the kanamycin resistance gene *neo*, with its native promoter P_{neo}.

According, the two plasmids Bsuc_PL87 and Bsuc_PL88 were equipped with 1500 bp long sequences from the 5' upstream and the 3' downstream non-coding region of *DD0789*, which both flanked the 943 bp long $P_{neo}neo$ DNA sequence, obtained from a pSEVA vector via PCR. The construct was cloned into the linearized (*ApaI*) vectors Bsuc_PL87 and Bsuc_PL88, which yielded the vectors Bsuc_PL94 and Bsuc_PL95, respectively. After plasmid validation and purification, strain engineering was conducted. The transformation yielded many clones, but only one blue colony was obtained for Bsuc_PL94 (**Figure 4.6 A**) and for Bsuc_PL95 (**Figure 4.6 B**), respectively, out of about 558 total clones.

The small percentage (0.4 %) of positive clones demonstrates the benefit of the screening for strain engineering in *B. succiniciproducens*. The two blue clones, apparently positive, were streaked. Subsequently, three individual blue colonies were tested using 5'-3'-PCR with the primer pairs P73+74 and P75+76 (**Figure 4.6 C**). It was shown that all individual colonies contained a 5' integration (P73+74) of the $P_{neo}neo$ DNA sequence, which was indicated by an observed PCR amplicon at around 2500 bp (**Figure 4.6 Lane A-F**). When wild type colonies were screened, an amplicon of about 3000 bp was detected, which comprised the native *DD0789* gene (**Figure *4.6* Lanes G-I**). Compared to the 3' integration screening (P75+76), no significant differences between the clones (**Figure 4.6 Lanes K-P**) and the wild type (**Figure 4.6 Lanes Q-S**) were observed. The negative controls (**Figure *4.6* Lane J and T**), containing water instead of DNA template, showed no contamination of the reaction.

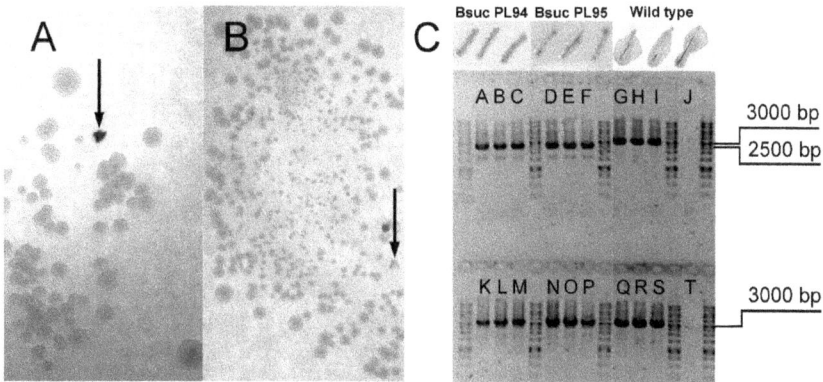

Figure 4.6. Results of *B. succiniciproducens* DD3ΔΔ*lacZ* transformation with Bsuc_PL94 and Bsuc_PL95. During the transformation procedure, electroporated cells were plated on buffered BHI agar, containing chloramphenicol (5 µg mL^{-1}) and X-gal (80 µg mL^{-1}). Transformation with Bsuc_PL94 yielded one blue colony which indicated vector integration into the genome (**A**). Also transformation with Bsuc_PL95 created one blue colony (**B**), out of about 558 clones. The blue colonies were streaked and three individual clones were screened via PCR (**C**) comprising Bsuc_PL94 and Bsuc_PL95 recombinants and the wild type. First recombination in 5' (Lanes A-J) and 3' (Lanes K-T) direction was tested by PCR using the primer pairs P73+74 and P75+76, respectively. Negative controls (Lane J+T) were conducted using demineralized water instead of DNA template. The gel comprised 1 % agarose using a 1 kb DNA ladder for determination of product size. Original gel is added to the appendix (**Figure 6.1**).

It can be concluded that the integration of the used vectors was proven successfully by use of the blue-white screening. The obtained blue clones exhibited the desired recombination, which was confirmed by PCR screening. As shown, the blue-white screening method was functional in *B. succiniciproducens* DD3ΔΔ*lacZ* to facilitate and support the identification of recombinants.

Further strain engineering aimed at the vector excision in a second recombination event. Again, the blue-white screening should highlight recombinants. Therefore, two positive clones containing the first recombination round were cultivated for 48 h in BHI medium without selection pressure to initiate the second recombination event. They were then plated in a dilution series on buffered BHI agar plates without chloramphenicol, but with 80 µg mL^{-1} X-gal (**Figure 4.7**). In sum, 18 white clones were obtained. These colonies were patched on buffered BHI, without chloramphenicol, containing X-gal for further examination using PCR (**Figure 4.8 A**). As control, blue colonies were patched additionally.

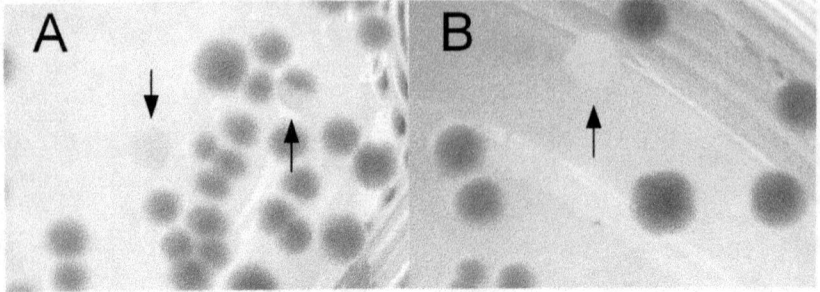

Figure 4.7. Second recombinant clone screening of *B. succiniciproducens* DD3ΔΔ*lacZ*Δ*DD0789-neo* using blue-white technique. Two positive clones of each recombinant strain *B. succiniciproducens* DD3ΔΔ*lacZ* containing the vectors were cultivated for 48 h in BHI without chloramphenicol. Subsequently, each culture broth was diluted serially 1:100000 and plated on buffered BHI agar plates containing 80 µg mL^{-1} X-gal. The Bsuc_PL94 strain (**A**), yielded 8 white clones, depicting potentially the strain *B. succiniciproducens* DD3ΔΔ*lacZ*Δ*DD0789-neo* or the wild type. Using the Bsuc_PL95 strain (**B**), 10 white clones were found. All 18 white clones were transferred on buffered BHI containing 80 µg mL^{-1} X-gal. Blue clones were also transferred as control. Further examination was conducted using PCR.

The PCR 5' screening with the primer pair P73+74 underlined the functionality of the blue-white screening. The 18 white clones comprised 5 clones which contained the desired Δ*DD0789*::P$_{neo}$*neo* genotype, designated as the *B. succiniciproducens* DD3ΔΔ*lacZ*Δ*DD0789-neo* strain (**Figure 4.8 Lanes 1, 13, 15, 16 and 18**). The remaining 13 clones exhibited the wild type PCR amplicon at about 3000 bp.

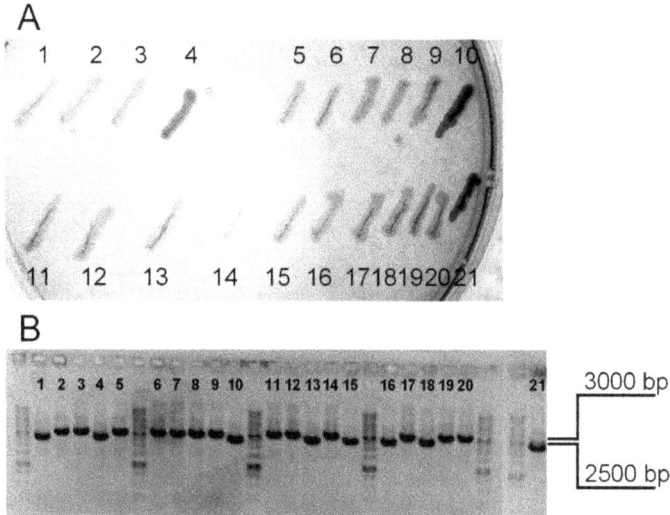

Figure 4.8. Validation of second recombinant clones of B. succiniciproducens DD3ΔΔlacZΔDD0789-neo using blue-white technique and PCR screening. The obtained clones (**A**) were screened by PCR with the 5' screening primer pair P73+74 (**B**). Screening revealed the success of the vector excision from the genome. At least, five out of 18 clones showed the deletion of DD0789, namely clone #1, #13, #15, #16 and #18. The new strain was designated as B. succiniciproducens DD3ΔΔlacZΔDD0789-neo. The results are emphasized by comparison to the control clones #4, #10 and #21, which turn blue and contain the plasmid and consequently the deletion of DD0789. Detection of amplicons were obtained by agarose gel electrophoresis. The gel comprised 1 % agarose using a 1 kb DNA ladder for determination of product size. Original gel is added to the appendix (**Figure 6.2**).

Additionally, it was tested if the B. succiniciproducens DD3ΔΔlacZΔDD0789-neo clones, containing the $P_{neo}neo$ modification, were viable on buffered BHI agar plates containing 10 µg mL^{-1} kanamycin (**Figure 4.9 A**). As control, a B. succiniciproducens DD3ΔΔlacZ clone and a blue clone, containing the Bsuc_PL94 or Bsuc_PL95 plasmid, were tested each. To prove clone viability, the same clones were patched on a non-selection agar plate (**Figure 4.9 B**). Obviously, all clones of B. succiniciproducens DD3ΔΔlacZΔDD0789-neo grew well on kanamycin, proving functionality of the genomic copy of the neo gene. In contrast, the non-modified B. succiniciproducens DD3ΔΔlacZ cells showed impaired growth. Surplus, the blue B. succiniciproducens DD3ΔΔlacZ clones containing the plasmid and though the kanamycin resistance gene, grew as well as the B. succiniciproducens DD3ΔΔlacZΔDD0789-neo clones, but showed the blue color. To sum it up, the blue-white selection screening was found suitable for genetic engineering of B. succiniciproducens.

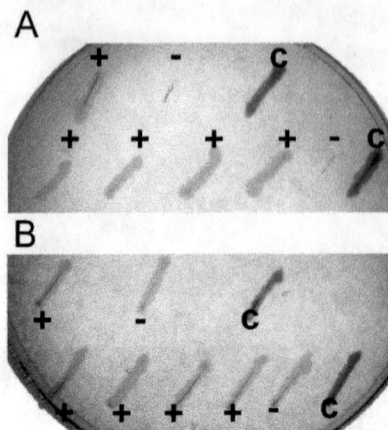

Figure 4.9. Growth test of *B. succiniciproducens* DD3ΔΔ*lacZ*Δ*DD0789-neo* on kanamycin. To test the functionality of the integrated kanamycin resistance gene (*neo*), the obtained clones were patched on buffered BHI agar plates containing 10 µg mL^{-1} kanamycin and 80 µg mL^{-1} X-gal (**A**) and buffered BHI agar plates containing 80 µg mL^{-1} X-gal (**B**). It was shown that all clones containing the knockout and the *neo* gene, indicated by a **plus**, grew on kanamycin. All wild type clones, indicated by a **minus** did not grow on kanamycin. The positive control clones, indicated by a **c**, which contained the plasmid and surplus the *neo* gene, grew as well and showed blue color.

The applicability of the new method was demonstrated by the successful deletion of the *DD0789* gene and the functional integration of the kanamycin resistance gene *neo* into the *DD0789* gene locus. For future strain construction, this technique can reduce costs and time effort.

4.2.5 Deletion of the gene *DD0789* impairs growth on sucrose

The deletion of the *DD0789* gene and the subsequent inactivation of the sucrose ptsG protein in *B. succiniciproducens* was now validated. Therefore, living cells of the parent strain and the deletion strain were used for inoculation of minimal medium containing glucose, fructose and sucrose, respectively. The growth was observed by measuring the optical density (OD$_{600}$) after 24 h of anaerobic cultivation (**Figure 4.10**). The knockout strain showed impaired growth on sucrose. Nevertheless, growth on glucose and fructose was still possible, in a similar manner compared to the parent strain. This experiment proved that the functional deletion of *DD0789* and the inactivation of the corresponding sucrose ptsG protein was successful.

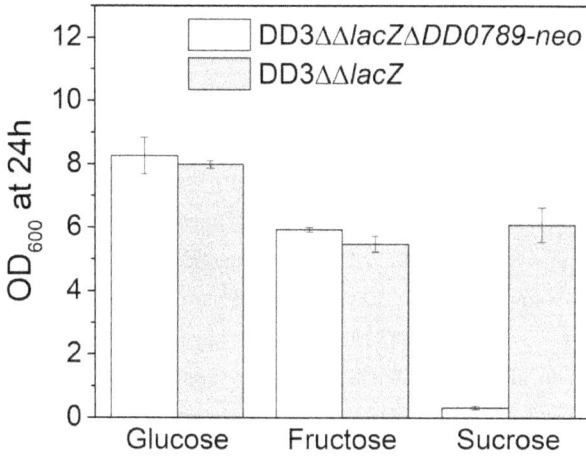

Figure 4.10. Growth ability of *B. succiniciproducens* **DD3ΔΔ*lacZ*Δ*DD0789-neo* and its parent strain on glucose, fructose and sucrose.** Optical density (OD_{600}) of the culture broth was measured after 24 h of anaerobic (CO_2) cultivation in minimal medium. The measured value is corrected for the inoculation optical density. The data represent means and deviation of duplicates.

4.2.6 Validation of functionality of *neo* gene integration into the genome

In order to prove the expression of the integrated *neo* gene and the functionality of the translated Neo protein, a screening experiment, using varied kanamycin concentrations was conducted. Therefore, a miniaturized and parallelized bioreactor system was used. The parent strain *B. succiniciproducens* DD3ΔΔ*lacZ* and the constructed strain *B. succiniciproducens* DD3ΔΔ*lacZ*Δ*DD0789-neo* were grown in BHI medium supplemented with 10 g L^{-1} glucose and additionally, 0, 2, 5, 10, 15, 20, 35 and 50 µg mL^{-1} of kanamycin (**Figure 4.11**).

In comparison, a significant difference in the growth behavior was observable. The parent strain was significantly affected, already at low kanamycin concentration (**Figure 4.11 A**). When 20 µg mL^{-1} of kanamycin was supplemented, only 17 % (0.14 h^{-1}) of the native growth rate (0.82 h^{-1}) was preserved. The addition of 35 µg mL^{-1} kanamycin stopped the growth almost completely. This concentration is defined as the minimal inhibitory concentration (MIC) for *B. succiniciproducens* on kanamycin.

In contrast, the mutant strain showed an enhanced resistance against the antibiotic (**Figure 4.11 B**). Here, 76 % (0.61 h^{-1}) of the maximum growth rate (0.81 h^{-1}) was still preserved at 20 µg mL^{-1} kanamycin.

A similar behavior was observed for *B. succiniciproducens* DD3ΔΔ*lacZ*Δ*DD0789-neo* when the optical density was considered (**Figure 4.11 C**). Again, 78 % of the reference value was reached, when 20 µg mL^{-1} of kanamycin was supplemented. This was significantly higher than the parent strain, which reached only 10 % of the unaffected OD_{620} under these conditions. Interestingly, almost 50 % of the maximum growth was preserved at 35 µg mL^{-1}, a level that affected the parent strain strongly. This provides evidence that the expression of the heterologous *neo* gene is possible in *B. succiniciproducens* and that the Neo protein is functional. This expands the toolbox for strain engineering, enabling counter selection on kanamycin, beside the commonly used chloramphenicol. When literature is considered, an almost similar selection concentration (25 µg mL^{-1}) was used recently in the relative bacterium *M. succiniciproducens* (Lee et al., 2006).

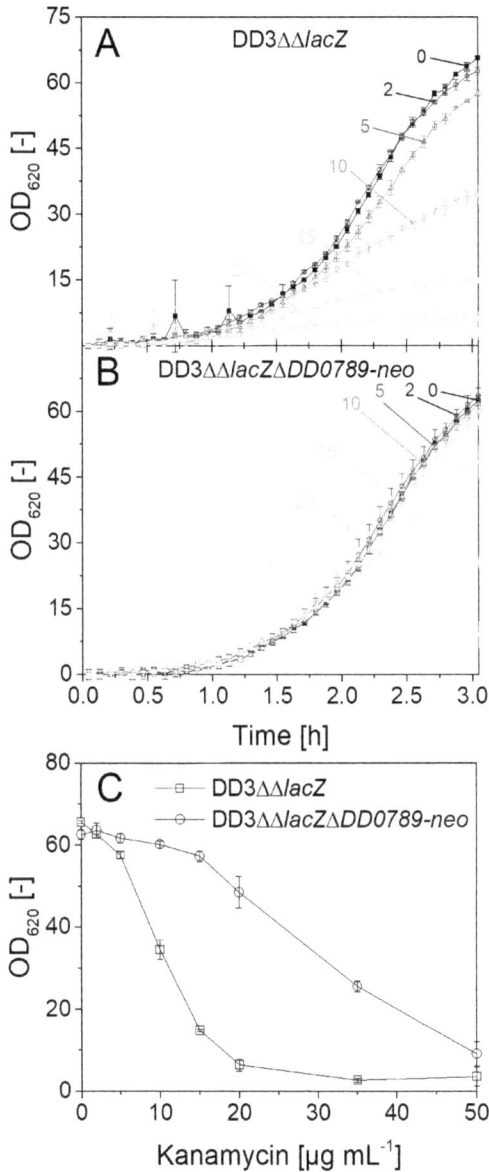

Figure 4.11. Growth impairment of *B. succiniciproducens* DD3ΔΔ*lacZ*Δ*DD0789-neo* and its parent strain induced by kanamycin. The cells were grown aerobically in BHI medium supplemented with 10 g L⁻¹ of glucose. Additionally, 2, 5, 10, 15, 20, 35 and 50 µg mL⁻¹ of kanamycin were added to the medium. Cultivation was conducted in a miniaturized and parallelized bioreactor system. Optical density at 620 nm (OD₆₂₀) was measured. The data represent three biological replicates with means and standard deviation.

As shown, the knockout of the sucrose ptsG was achieved successfully. The strain engineering was shown to be fast and efficient. Screening steps, normally conducted using PCR, can be reduced. Additionally, the successful deletion was shown by growth impairment of the mutant strain on sucrose. Surplus, the functionality of the integrated *neo* gene was successful demonstrated, which increased the resistance of *B. succiniciproducens* against kanamycin. This engineered technique was now available for metabolic engineering of *B. succiniciproducens*.

4.2.7 Evaluation of native promoter strength to support heterologous gene expression in *Basfia succiniciproducens*

Beside successful implementation of engineering strategies for *B. succiniciproducens*, we know very little about the expression of heterologous proteins in this bacterium. In particular, we lack knowledge on suitable promoters that can be exploited to achieve high expression level. As shown for various microorganisms, the strength of the promoter is one of the most important elements to control expression level (De Mey et al., 2007; Keasling, 2010; Rytter et al., 2014). So far, most studies with rumen bacteria describe their natural ability to produce succinic acid and the construction of superior mutants mainly involved the deletion of genes, rather than the integration of novel ones (Becker et al., 2013; Choi et al., 2016; Pateraki et al., 2016). Accordingly, our knowledge on suitable promoters for high-level expression of heterologous genes in rumen bacteria is rather limited, whereas it is even missing for *B. succiniciproducens* (Jang et al., 2007).

For this purpose, a GFP-coupled screening system was established to determine the strength of native promoters of *B. succiniciproducens*. The aerobic test conditions allowed to directly use common GFP as a reporter, which requires oxygen for maturation (Cormack et al., 1996). In a first screening campaign, promoters which regulate apparently active pathways to prominent by-products, i.e. formate (*pflA*, *pflD*) and lactate (*ldhA*), were selected as potential candidates. In addition, the housekeeping promoter of the superoxide dismutase gene (*sodC*) was chosen, due to its beneficial properties for high-level expression in other bacteria (Becker et al., 2007).

Each promoter was amplified from the genome sequence of *B. succiniciproducens*, and was then cloned in front of the GFP reporter gene on the episomal plasmid pJFF224. The derived plasmids were namely Bsuc_PL8 ($P_{pflD}GFP$), Bsuc_PL9 ($P_{pflA}GFP$), Bsuc_PL10 ($P_{ldhA}GFP$) and Bsuc_PL11 ($P_{sodC}GFP$). The associated strains of *B. succiniciproducens* DD3 were used for expression analysis. For each promoter, fluorescence was proportional to the cell concentration over time, indicating a steady expression level during the cultivation of the reporter strains (**Figure 4.12 A - D**). This allowed quantification of the specific promoter activity from the slope of the obtained correlation (**Figure 4.12 E**). In direct comparison, the *pflD* promoter showed the highest expression, followed by P_{pflA}, which exhibited about 60 % of P_{pflD} activity. Only relatively weak expression was observed for P_{sodC} and P_{ldhA}. The promoters of pyruvate formate lyase (P_{pflA}, P_{pflD}) enabled strongest expression within the tested set of homologous candidates. The promoter is efficiently induced by pyruvate (Sawers and Böck, 1988; Yang et al., 2001). This is promising, because pyruvate and pyruvate-based by-products were observed in aerobic metabolism in *B. succiniciproducens*, as shown previously (**Figure 4.2**). The latter can help to stimulate gene expression in engineered hosts regarding pyruvate-based production pathways under control of the *pflD* promoter.

Surprisingly, the *sodC* promoter, previously found highly active in gram-positive *C. glutamicum* (Becker et al., 2011), was not that active, as one might have expected. Obviously, *B. succiniciproducens* requires specifically selected promoters, similar to what is known for other microorganisms (Jang et al., 2007; Rytter et al., 2014).

So far, nothing is known about the activity of heterologous promoters in *B. succiniciproducens*. Thus, a derivative (P_{EM7*}) of the commonly known strong and constitutive P_{EM7} promoter (Drocourt et al., 2007) was tested randomly. This derivative was derived by random mutagenesis and found highly active in *P. putida* (Rogsch, 2015). Surprisingly, this modified promoter was also active in *B. succiniciproducens*. A distinct experiment revealed, that P_{EM7*} enabled an almost 290 % increase in GFP expression by use of the established screening system (**Figure 4.13**). This is a valuable proof, that also heterologous promoters can be used in *B. succiniciproducens* to engage heterologous gene expression. The latter broadens furthermore the molecular toolbox for strain engineering of *B. succiniciproducens*.

It can be concluded that the identified set of promoters is a basis for directed strain engineering regarding heterologous gene expression. Especially the P_{pflD} and P_{EM7*}

promoters seemed to support efficient expression. The P_{pflD} promoter is supposed to be efficiently used for further strain engineering of *B. succiniciproducens* for the production of the pyruvate-based product L-alanine. Without doubt, the set of newly identified promoters might also be useful for application in other rumen bacteria.

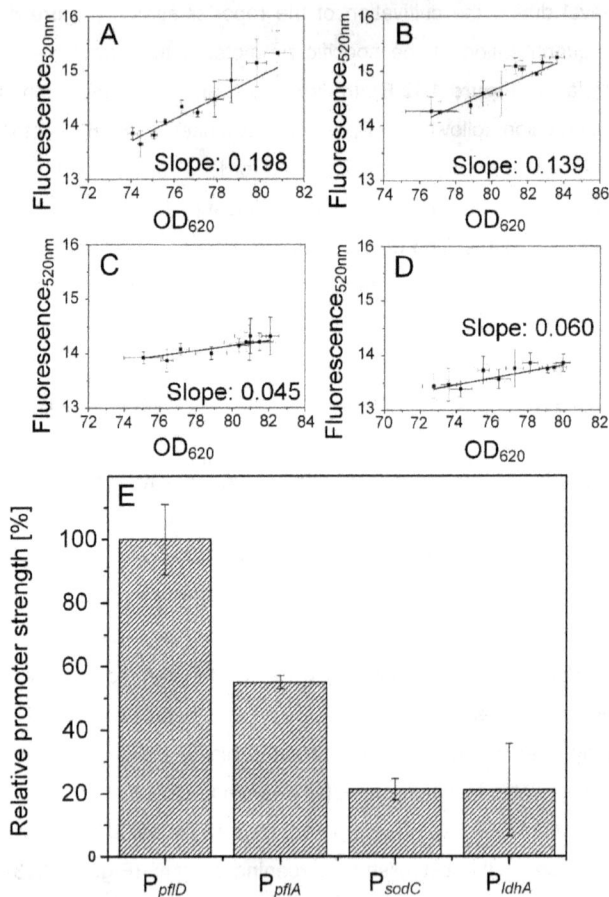

Figure 4.12. Expression strength of *B. succiniciproducens* promoters, using green fluorescent protein (GFP) as reporter. Correlation between on-line recorded fluorescence at 520 nm and cell concentration at OD_{620} during growth of *B. succiniciproducens* DD3 reporter strains, used for estimation of specific promoter strength: DD3 + Bsuc_PL8 containing $P_{pflD}GFP$ (**A**), DD3 + Bsuc_PL9 containing $P_{pflA}GFP$ (**B**), DD3 + Bsuc_PL10 containing $P_{sodC}GFP$ (**C**), DD3 + Bsuc_PL11 containing $P_{ldhA}GFP$ (**D**). Specific promoter activity, normalized to the strongest promoter, which was set to 100 % (**E**). Mean values and standard deviations reflect three biological replicates. The data are corrected for basal fluorescence of *B. succiniciproducens* DD3, carrying the empty plasmid pJFF224.

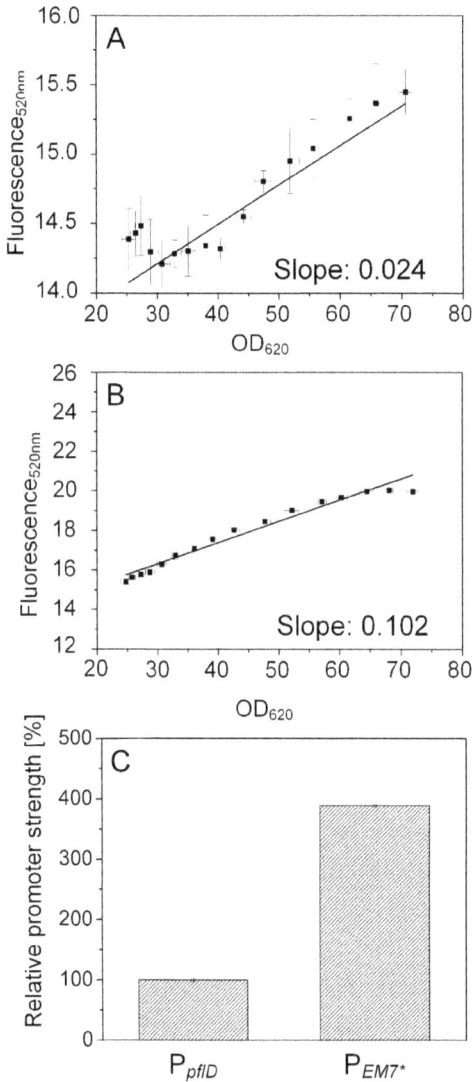

Figure 4.13. Expression strength of the heterologous *EM7** promoter, using green fluorescent protein (GFP) as reporter. On-line recorded fluorescence at 520 nm and cell concentration at OD_{620} was correlated during exponential growth of *B. succiniciproducens* DD3 reporter strains, used for estimation of specific promoter strength: DD3 + Bsuc_PL8 containing $P_{pflD}GFP$ (**A**), DD3 + Bsuc_PL104 containing P_{EM7^*}-GFP (**B**). Specific promoter activity, normalized to the known strong P_{pflD} promoter, which was set to 100 % (**C**). Mean values and standard deviations reflect three biological replicates. The data are corrected for basal fluorescence of *B. succiniciproducens* DD3, carrying the empty plasmid pJFF224.

4.3 Application of *Basfia succiniciproducens* for ʟ-alanine production

In a recent study, the recombinant strain *B. succiniciproducens* ALA-1 was engineered for ʟ-alanine production (Fabarius, 2013). By homologous recombination, a heterologous alanine dehydrogenase (*alaD*) from *G. stearothermophilus* XL65-6 under control of the previously identified strong *pflD* promoter, was introduced in the *pflD* gene locus. This gene was codon-optimized for *B. succiniciproducens* to stabilize its expression. *B. succiniciproducens* DD3 was used as the parent strain, which contains the *ldhA* and *pflD* gene knockout. These knockouts eliminate the production of lactate and formate. The latter enhanced the production of the alanine precursor pyruvate and derived by-products (Becker et al., 2013). This novel alanine producer strain was now examined in a complex medium on glucose to assess its physiology.

4.3.1 Aerobic physiology of a novel alanine overproducer

Taken to the shake flask, the strain grew from early on and consumed the glucose rapidly within 12 h. The recombinant strain produced, after a short lag phase, 0.7 ± 0.2 g L^{-1} ʟ-alanine (**Figure 4.14**) within 12 h, whereas the parent strain *B. succiniciproducens* DD3 did not accumulate the desired product in significant amounts (**Figure 4.2**). The overall product yield of 43.3 ± 10 mg$_{alanine}$ g^{-1}$_{glucose}$ was comparably low. Most of the carbon was channeled into acetate (5.2 ± 0.2 g L^{-1}) owing to the examined conditions. Additionally, 2.1 ± 0.8 g L^{-1} succinate were produced.

Subsequent measurements of enzyme activities in both strains (**Figure 4.15**) revealed that *B. succiniciproducens* ALA-1 exhibited a specific alanine dehydrogenase activity of 280 ± 76 mU mg^{-1} during amination of pyruvate. As assumed, alanine dehydrogenase reaction was obviously reversible, as indicated by the deamination reaction of alanine combined with NAD$^+$ during enzyme assay tests. Here, an enzyme activity of 43 ± 4 mU mg^{-1} was determined. The control strain did not exhibit activity (< 0.1 mU mg^{-1}) in both reaction directions, as expected, due to lack of a native alanine dehydrogenase in the genome. Furthermore, both strains revealed similar activity for G6P dehydrogenase, analyzed as positive control (250 ± 43 mU mg^{-1} for DD3 and 193 ± 25 mU mg^{-1} for ALA-1).

To exclude the origin of the produced alanine from the complex fraction of the medium, a labelling experiment was designed. Therefore, naturally labelled glucose was replaced by [$^{13}C_6$] glucose, followed by GC/MS analysis of ʟ-alanine, harvested from the culture broth at the end of the cultivation. The fully labeled [$^{13}C_3$] L-alanine mass isotopomer was the dominating fraction, verifying its *De-novo* synthesis from glucose (**Figure 4.16**).

Taken together, the results emphasize that a novel alanine producer was established. The next steps should examine its production capacities through process engineering.

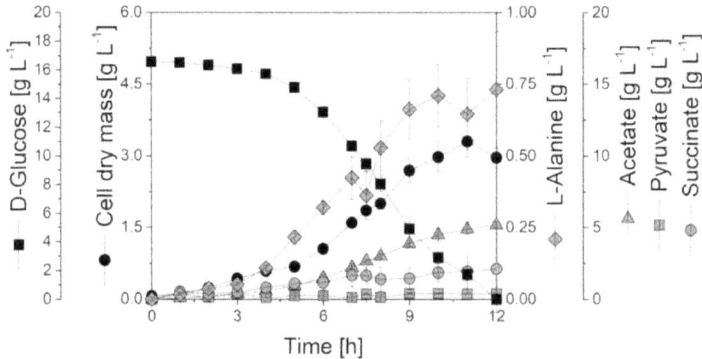

Figure 4.14. Aerobic cultivation physiology of *B. succiniciproducens* DD3 ALA-1 in shake flask. The newly constructed alanine overproducer formed 0.70 ± 0.2 g L^{-1} of alanine in 12 h. Measurement of organic acids, sugars and amino acids was conducted using HPLC. The data represent three independent replicates with means and deviation.

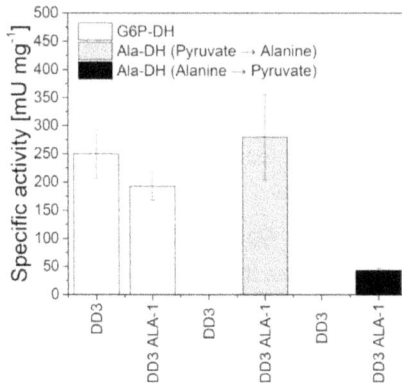

Figure 4.15. Detection of alanine dehydrogenase activity in *B. succiniciproducens* DD3 and DD3 ALA-1. To prove the expression of alanine dehydrogenase in the novel engineered strain DD3 ALA-1, enzyme assays were conducted. Activity of AlaD protein was shown in the modified strain DD3 ALA-1, whereas no activity was measured in the parent strain DD3. As positive control, glucose 6-phosphate dehydrogenase was assayed, which showed comparable activities for both strains. All data represent three independent replicates with means and deviation.

59

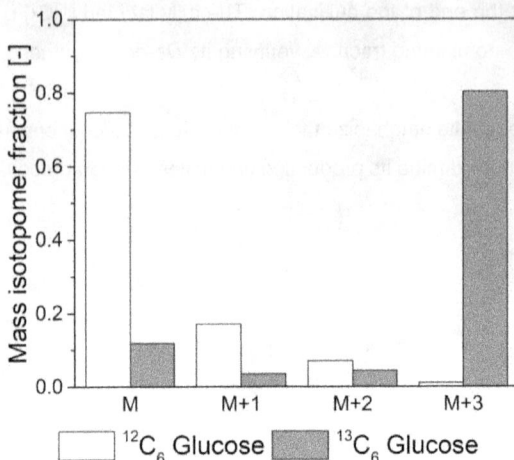

Figure 4.16. GC-MS analysis of TBDMS derivatized alanine from the culture supernatant of
B. succiniciproducens **ALA-1 grown on naturally labelled glucose (white bars) and on [$^{13}C_6$]**
glucose (grey bars). M+0, M+1, M+2, M+3 reflect the monoisotopic, the single labelled, the double
labelled, and the triple labelled mass isotopomer, respectively. The measurement was conducted on the
ion cluster *m/z* 260-263, which represents a fragment ion of the analyte that contains the entire carbon
skeleton of alanine.

4.3.2 Metabolic overflow at the pyruvate-node impairs efficient alanine production

Taken to an aerobic fed-batch environment in lab scale bioreactors, alanine production
from glucose using *B. succiniciproducens* ALA-1 could be increased to 7.2 ± 1.0 g L^{-1}
within 36 h (**Figure 4.17**). This was accompanied by strong formation of acetate and
pyruvate, which impaired overall production performance significantly. The process
was operated as a fed-batch with an initial batch phase and pulse-wise feeding,
coupled to the level of dissolved oxygen via the on-line signal of the oxygen probe.
The cells grew from early on and reached a cell concentration of about 11 ± 0.1 g L^{-1}
after 5 hours, accompanied by a μ_{max} of 0.74 ± 0.01 h^{-1}. A single feed pulse after
3 hours, triggered by a sudden rise in the dissolved oxygen signal, led to a transiently
increased glucose level, but did not negatively impact growth. About 2.5 g L^{-1} of
L-alanine was produced during the initial batch phase. Up to this point of the
fermentation, acetate was the dominating by-product and reached about
17.6 ± 0.4 g L^{-1}.

With depletion of glucose after 5 hours, cell growth stopped and the automated feed addition was initiated. The entry into glucose limitation caused an interesting switch in the growth mode. For a short period of about 2 hours, excreted pyruvate and acetate, together with L-alanine, were taken up by the cells again, likely to maintain high carbon influx. Subsequently, L-alanine production was re-activated and continued on a high level until the end of the process, when the final titer was reached. Interestingly, acetate accumulation ceased shortly after cell growth had stopped and the acetate level remained constant further on. Pyruvate was secreted for a longer time up to 12.0 ± 0.5 g L^{-1}, but finally also stopped, leading to a purely L-alanine producing process.

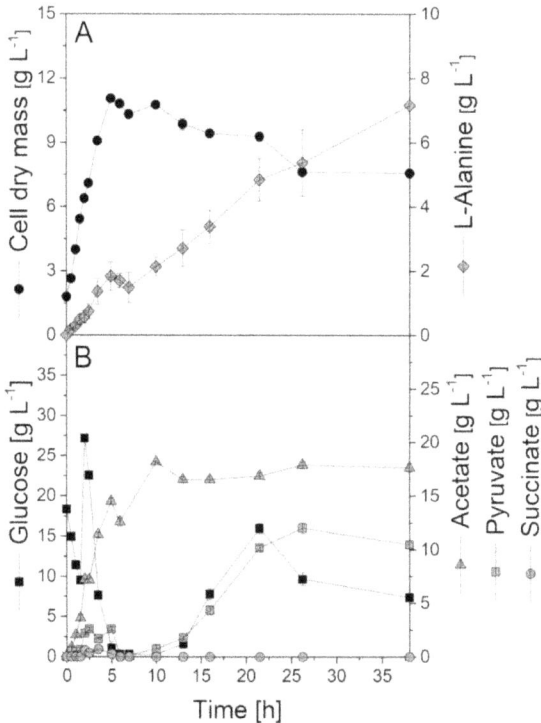

Figure 4.17. Aerobic fed-batch production of L-alanine by *B. succiniciproducens* ALA-1 from glucose. An initial batch phase was followed by a carbon limiting feed phase via dissolved oxygen based feeding. A pure alanine production process (**A**) was observed, yielding 7.2 ± 1.0 g L^{-1} alanine. Predominantly, acetate and pyruvate were produced (**B**). The data shown represent biological duplicates with mean values and deviations.

4.3.3 Screening of industrial relevant substrates under different process conditions

To determine the alanine production capabilities of the strain, a set of experiments now investigated the impact of the carbon source under different production conditions. In addition to glucose, fructose, sucrose, xylose and glycerol were tested (**Figure 4.18**). *B. succiniciproducens* ALA1 was grown aerobically on the different substrates (**Figure 4.18 A**). Interestingly, the final titer for L-alanine was highest on xylose. The achieved amount (1.7 ± 0.1 g L^{-1}) exceeded that observed for glucose by more than 140 %. In comparison, fructose and sucrose led to only weak formation of L-alanine, whereas the performance on glycerol was similar to glucose-grown cells. Acetate formation was rather unaffected by the carbon source.

Subsequently, the different carbon sources were also tested under anaerobic conditions. Since several studies revealed superior performances under oxygen deprivation (Jojima et al., 2010; Yamamoto et al., 2012; Zhang et al., 2007; Zhou et al., 2015), a N$_2$ atmosphere was applied (**Figure 4.18 B**). Generally, L-alanine production was significantly higher as compared to aerobic conditions whereas biomass yield decreased substantially. Coherently, acetate formation was strongly lowered, indicating a carbon re-direction from acetate to the product, and also a connection between growth and acetate production, as observed before. Again, xylose enabled the highest product titer (7.9 ± 0.1 g L^{-1}), which was more than 30 % higher than that on glucose (5.8 ± 0.1 g L^{-1}). Fructose and sucrose also led to high levels of L-alanine, but the production was slightly lower than that achieved on the pentose. Glycerol was found rather non suitable under these conditions, due to missing growth of the cultures under the applied conditions. On this carbon source, the mutant produced below 1.0 ± 0.0 g L^{-1} L-alanine.

Apparently, xylose appeared to be a superior carbon source for alanine production, as indicated by the results. Additionally, the strong influence of the anaerobic environment led furthermore to an improved alanine titer of 370 %, when aerobic and anaerobic conditions on xylose were compared directly. The excellent performance on xylose is highly promising, as the pentose can be obtained from lignocellulosic biomass (Takisawa et al., 2017). Xylose is regarded as the second abundant sugar in lignocellulose after glucose, and is the major component accounting for more than 30 % and 90 % in cellulosic and hemicellulosic hydrolysates, respectively (Van Dyk and Pletschke, 2012).

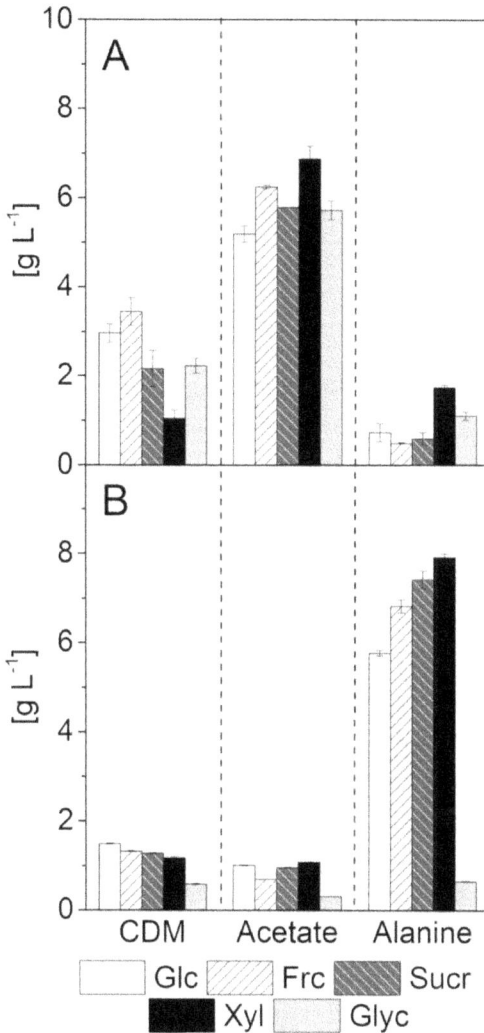

Figure 4.18. Impact of the carbon source on L-alanine production in engineered B. succiniciproducens ALA-1. The data shown represent final values, obtained after 24 h of cultivation under aerobic conditions (**A**) and after 48 h under anaerobic conditions (N₂ atmosphere) (**B**). In all cases, the initially added substrate (15 g L⁻¹ glucose (glc), fructose (frc), sucrose (sucr), xylose (xyl) and glycerol (glyc)) was completely consumed (except anaerobic glycerol test due to lacking growth) at the time point of sampling. The data represent biological duplicates with mean values and deviations.

4.3.4 Optimization of xylose-based L-alanine production using different gas atmospheres

Xylose was studied in more detail, due to its superior efficiency for L-alanine production. Different culture conditions were compared to identify the most promising set-up. Grown aerobically, *B. succiniciproducens* ALA-1 completely consumed xylose in about 24 h and accumulated L-alanine to a final concentration of 1.7 ± 0.1 g L^{-1} (**Figure 4.19 A**). Acetate was still the main product (6.4 ± 0.2 g L^{-1}). In addition, small amounts of succinate were formed (1.3 ± 0.2 g L^{-1}). Biomass was formed, particularly during the initial phase of the cultivation. The production was next operated as a two-stage process in order to combine the good growth performance of the aerobic cultures during the first hours (**Figure 4.19 A**) with the good L-alanine production performance under anaerobic conditions (**Figure 4.18 B**).

In two alternative settings, the initial aerobic growth phase was coupled to a second production phase under pure CO_2 and under pure N_2 as gas phase (**Figure 4.19 B + C**). The initial growth phase indeed allowed fast biomass formation and xylose consumption. Acetate was inherently formed as a side product and reached a concentration of about 2.5 ± 0.1 g L^{-1} at the end of the growth phase after 10 hours. Slight formation of alanine was observed during this phase as well.

After the switch to the CO_2 atmosphere, cells continued to consume xylose, but now exhibited a strongly changed production behavior: L-alanine accumulation increased significantly, whereas acetate formation stopped immediately (**Figure 4.19 B**). After 36 hours, the final L-alanine titer was 3.1 ± 0.0 g L^{-1}. Driven by the CO_2 atmosphere, succinate formation was relatively strong and the compound reached a final level of 9.3 ± 0.4 g L^{-1}. Increased availability of CO_2 is regarded as major driver of phosphoenolpyruvate carboxykinase (Kim et al., 2009) and subsequent anaplerotic fueling of the reductive TCA cycle leading to the observed succinate accumulation. In contrast, pyruvate was completely abolished as side product. The concentration of acetate did not change during the production phase and thus seemed to be coupled to the aerobic conditions of the initial growth phase. Underlined by the 80 % increased product titer, the overall production characteristics were improved compared to the aerobic process.

The cultures, incubated under N_2 during the production phase, showed an even better performance (**Figure 4.19 C**). Under these conditions, the mutant achieved a final L-alanine titer of 6.4 ± 0.2 g L^{-1}. The elevated formation of the amino acid was linked to a reduction in succinate formation (6.9 ± 0.8 g L^{-1}) by 25 %. This example demonstrated that it is possible to shift alanine to a main product of the metabolism of *B. succiniciproducens* ALA-1.

These results demonstrate successfully the shift of the product spectrum from acetate and succinate to predominantly alanine by using aerobic conditions, CO_2 or N_2, respectively. Under commonly used growth conditions, i.e. glucose and elevated levels of CO_2, the recombinant strain *B. succiniciproducens* ALA-1 still produced L-alanine poorly, but rather showed the typically described strong accumulation of succinate instead. Selected rumen bacteria have been shown to secrete small traces of L-alanine, among other amino acids from sugars (Stevenson, 1978). Moreover, none of the studied strains so far exhibited significant overproduction of L-alanine or related carbon-three chemicals (Becker et al., 2013; Becker and Wittmann, 2012b; Choi et al., 2013; Choi et al., 2016; Schindler et al., 2014; Xi et al., 2013). The next step regarded lab scale bioreactor experiments to uncork the full potential of the investigated strain.

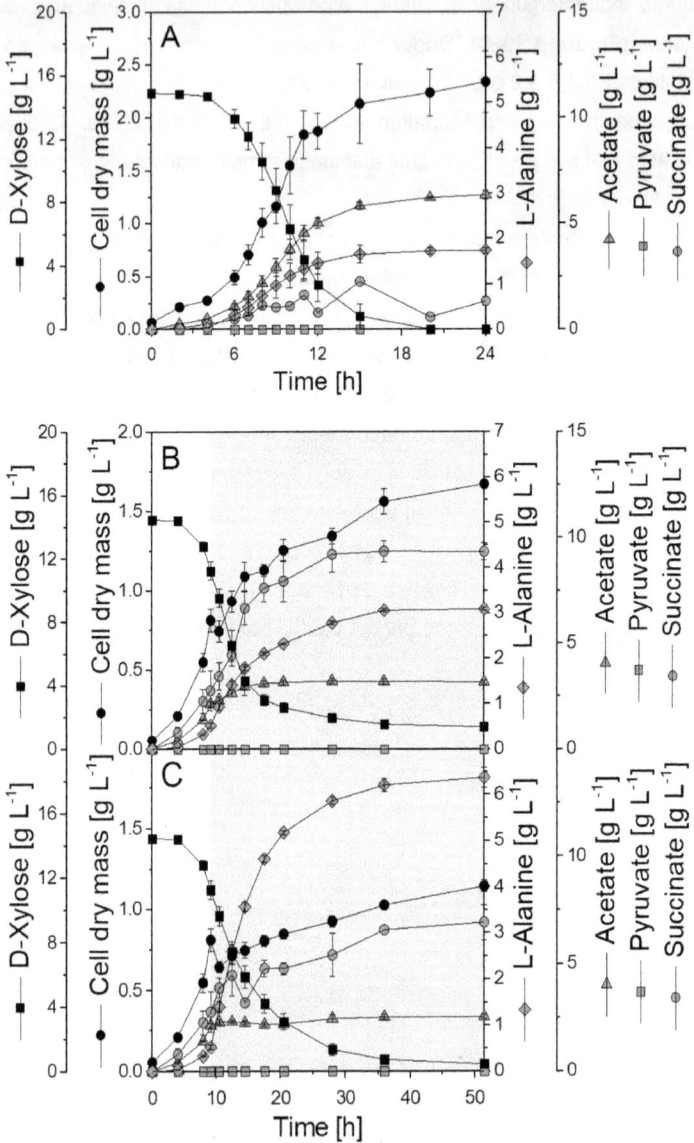

Figure 4.19. L-alanine production in engineered *B. succiniciproducens* ALA-1 from xylose. Aerobic conditions (**A**) were compared to a two-phase process with an initial aerobic growth phase, followed by an anaerobic production phase under a CO_2 atmosphere (**B**) and in a two-phase process with an initial aerobic growth phase, followed by an anaerobic production phase under a N_2 atmosphere (**C**). Data reflect mean values and deviations from three biological replicates.

4.3.5 Batch production of L-alanine from xylose under N_2 atmosphere

The production of alanine was next studied in lab scale bioreactors, operated in batch mode (**Figure 4.20**). In order to support process efficiency, cells were inoculated to a comparably high initial concentration of about 7.0 ± 0.2 g L^{-1} cell dry mass.

Under microaerobic conditions without gassing (**Figure 4.20 A-C**) *B. succiniciproducens* ALA-1 consumed xylose from early on and completely depleted the carbon source within only 3 hours. This was accompanied by rapid L-alanine production. After 3 h, a final titer of 25.2 ± 1.8 g L^{-1} was reached, matching a product yield of 0.49 ± 0.03 g$_{alanine}$ g$_{xylose}^{-1}$. The maximum specific productivity was 2.3 ± 0.0 g g^{-1} h^{-1}. During the incubation, the cell concentration remained rather constant. A fraction of the substrate carbon was channeled into acetate (2.6 ± 0.3 g L^{-1}) and into succinate (10.6 ± 0.6 g L^{-1}).

A strictly anaerobic atmosphere with N_2 gassing (**Figure 4.20 D-F**) was even better for production. The product titer (27.0 ± 2.2 g L^{-1}) and the product yield (0.60 ± 0.03 g g^{-1}) were substantially higher except the maximum specific productivity (1.9 ± 0.0 g g^{-1} h^{-1}). In addition, production was much more selective. The formation of succinate (6.5 ± 0.5 g L^{-1}) was reduced by 40 %, while the formation of acetate (0.54 ± 0.18 g L^{-1}) was diminished. Similar to the microaerobic process (**Table 4.2**), the conversion was completed within 3 h, whereby the cell concentration stayed relatively constant.

The developed strain achieved the excellent performance of a recent recombinant *E. coli* (Zhang et al., 2007). The basic producer *E. coli* XZ111 also expresses alanine dehydrogenase from a single genomic copy and lacks competing pathways to pyruvate-based by-products and therefore appears most straightforward for direct comparison of the two microbes. In batch culture, the titer (25 g L^{-1}) was 40 % higher for *B. succiniciproducens* ALA-1, as compared to the glucose-grown *E. coli* strain, and the overall specific productivity (2.3 g g^{-1} h^{-1}) surpassed the value by the *E. coli* producer more than twentyfold. Although significantly suppressed in cells, grown on xylose under N_2, the formation of succinate was not completely eliminated. This is one major reason for the suboptimal yield and remains to be addressed in future developments, as *E. coli* enables practically exclusive production of L-alanine. Low levels of formed lactate correspond to the methylglyoxal pathway (Grabar et al., 2006), because lactate dehydrogenase was deleted in the *B. succiniciproducens* ALA-1 genome, suggesting straightforward strain engineering.

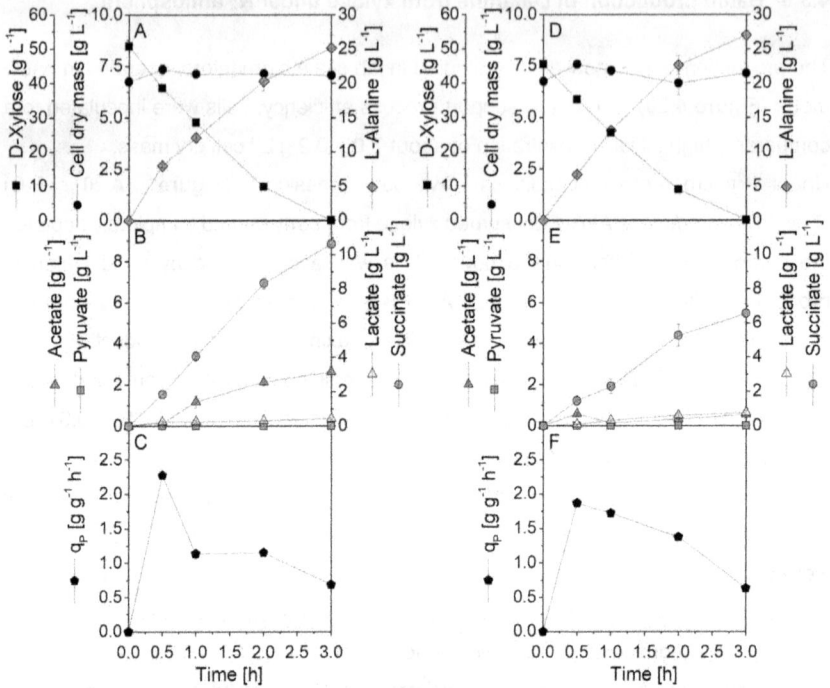

Figure 4.20. Batch production of L-alanine from xylose in lab-scale bioreactors using *B. succiniciproducens* ALA-1. Microaerobic conditions without gassing (**A-C**) and anaerobic conditions with N_2 gassing (**D-F**) were deployed. Data reflect mean values and deviations from two biological replicates.

4.3.6 Fed-batch production of L-alanine from xylose

Finally, the producing strain was evaluated in a fed-batch environment using again xylose as carbon source. A first setup coupled an initial aerobic batch phase for growth with a subsequent anaerobic feed phase (N_2) for production (**Figure 4.21 A-C**). The cells consumed xylose from early. After already 2 hours, the substrate level had decreased to about 6.0 ± 0.2 g L^{-1}, which then triggered the start of the feed and the switch in the gas supply from air to N_2. During this initial batch phase, a cell dry mass concentration of about 2.4 ± 0.2 g L^{-1} was reached. In addition, about 2.0 ± 0.0 g L^{-1} of L-alanine was produced. Growth was linked to the accumulation of acetate (3.5 ± 0.0 g L^{-1}) as observed previously. Immediately after the change in the cultivation mode, cell growth and acetate formation stopped. From the on-set of the feed addition until the very end of the process, the xylose level remained within the desired corridor between 5 and 15 g L^{-1}. Within 48 hours, 28.2 ± 2.0 g L^{-1} L-alanine was formed. The overall product yield was 0.50 ± 0.02 g g^{-1} and the maximum specific productivity was 1.7 ± 0.1 g g^{-1} h^{-1}. It was interesting to note that the different production phases had a strong impact on by-product formation. Succinate did not accumulate during the aerobic growth phase, but was formed after the switch to the anaerobic conditions. After about 9 hours, cells revealed a switch in their product spectrum. While succinate production slowed down significantly, small amounts of lactate and pyruvate were formed.

A second setup was designed as fully anaerobic process with N_2 supply (**Figure 4.21 D-F**). Here, *B. succiniciproducens* ALA-1 grew during the first 24 hours up to a cell dry mass concentration of 2.5 g ± 0.2 L^{-1}, which then remained constant until the end of the process. After 60 h, a final titer of 29.4 ± 2.4 g L^{-1} L-alanine was reached, corresponding to a product yield of 0.60 ± 0.1 g g^{-1}. The maximum specific production rate was 1.7 ± 0.2 g g^{-1} h^{-1}. Compared to batch processes, it was not possible to achieve higher titers by the fed-batch process. There seems to be a bottleneck hampering the alanine productivity of the cells in later process stages.

An overview over the conducted processes with *B. succiniciproducens* ALA-1 is summarized in **Table 4.2**. Given that additional rounds of metabolic engineering and strain evolution further improve performance, as impressively demonstrated for *E. coli* (Zhang et al., 2007), *B. succiniciproducens* ALA-1 exhibits highly promising potential to be further developed towards industrial L-alanine production.

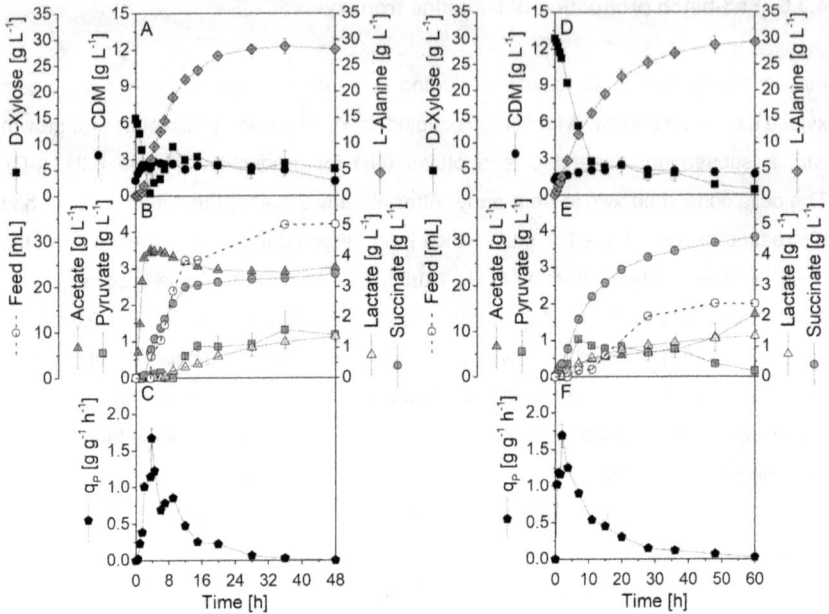

Figure 4.21. Fed-batch production of L-alanine from D-xylose using *B. succiniciproducens* ALA-1. One process design combined a dual-phase process with an initial aerobic batch phase, followed by an anaerobic production phase with N₂ gassing (**A-C**). Additionally, a two-stage process divided in the aerobic biomass preparation followed by a subsequent anaerobic process with N₂ gassing was used (**D-F**). The data shown represent biological duplicates with mean values and deviations. CDM, Cell dry mass.

Table 4.2. Production of L-alanine by *B. succiniciproducens* ALA-1 using batch and fed-batch production with xylose as the carbon source. The data given comprise the final L-alanine titer, the specific substrate uptake rate (q$_S$), the maximum specific L-alanine production rate (q$_{P, max}$), the maximum volumetric productivity (Q$_{P, max}$), and the product yield and reflect mean values and deviations from duplicates.

Substrate	Process	L-alanine [g L⁻¹]	q$_S$[a] [g g⁻¹ h⁻¹]	q$_{p, max}$ [g g⁻¹ h⁻¹]	Q$_{p, max}$[b] [g L⁻¹ h⁻¹]	Y$_{P/S}$[c] [g g⁻¹]
Xylose	Microaerobic batch	25.20 ± 1.84	2.41 ± 0.04	2.27 ± 0.01	8.40 ± 0.50	0.48 ± 0.04
Xylose	Anaerobic batch (N₂)	27.00 ± 2.20	2.19 ± 0.05	1.87 ± 0.04	9.00 ± 0.59	0.60 ± 0.05
Xylose	Aerobic batch, Anaerobic feed phase (N₂)	28.16 ± 2.00	2.1 ± 0.06	1.67 ± 0.14	0.59 ± 0.03	0.50 ± 0.02
Xylose	Anaerobic fed-batch (N₂)	29.35 ± 2.40	1.61 ± 0.09	1.69 ± 0.16	0.49 ± 0.03	0.60 ± 0.06

[a] The specific substrate uptake rate refers to the batch phase of each experiment
[b] The volumetric productivity refers to the mean value of the total process
[c] For the fed-batch processes, the yield refers to the value obtained during the feed phase

4.3.7 *Basfia succiniciproducens* ALA-1 is a promising strain for L-alanine production.

As shown, *B. succiniciproducens* ALA-1 was used as a host for L-alanine production. The double deletion mutant *B. succiniciproducens* Δ*ldhA* Δ*pflD*, previously designated *B. succiniciproducens* DD3, was selected as host, because it already exhibited the desired feature of lacking the pathways to major competing by-products (Becker et al., 2013; Scholten and Dägele, 2008). Rumen bacteria belonging to the *Pasteurellaceae* group, such as *M. succiniciproducens* (Hong et al., 2004), *A. succinogenes* (Guettler et al., 1999), and *B. succiniciproducens* (Kuhnert et al., 2010), are described as capnophilic microbes, which naturally use fumarate as the final electron acceptor and secrete succinate, while efficiently fixing CO_2. This results in enormous succinic acid yields up to 75 % even in wild types (Becker et al., 2013). Accordingly, research so far has focused to further explore this biosynthetic potential and breed strains for elevated production of succinic acid and other related carbon-four chemicals from the reductive TCA cycle (Becker et al., 2013; Choi et al., 2013; Choi et al., 2016; Pateraki et al., 2016; Salvachúa et al., 2016).

Interestingly, *B. succiniciproducens* excretes pyruvate-derived metabolites, when the pathways of the natural by-products lactate and formate are interrupted on genome level (Becker et al., 2013). Hence, beyond previous work, it was shown that the product spectrum of rumen bacteria can be significantly altered towards pyruvate-based products and that this relies on combined efforts of metabolic and bioprocess engineering. In particular, the expression of the used heterologous *alaD* gene had to be high enough to mediate sufficient enzymatic activity for alanine production. Here, the promoter of the pyruvate formate lyase was later found capable to enable the excellent performance of the created L-alanine producing strain under aerobic or either anaerobic conditions. The full metabolic potential of the strain was released, when cells were grown under N_2 gassing with the lignocellulose based substrate xylose. Gassing resulted in low levels of CO_2, as endogenously formed CO_2 was continuously stripped out of the culture resulting in lowered succinate production. This enhanced the availability of carbon for alanine formation drastically. Beyond L-alanine, the present findings open interesting possibilities to re-engineer *B. succiniciproducens* and related rumen bacteria for other carbon-three products of industrial relevance such as pyruvate (Zhu et al., 2008) and lactate (Tsuge et al., 2015), among others.

4.4 Metabolic engineering for β-alanine production

B. succiniciproducens is known as a strong succinate overproducer (Becker et al., 2013; Lange et al., 2017). Thus, further engineering to use this capability for other products derived from succinate or related precursors seemed promising. As example, the related succinate-producer *M. succiniciproducens* was re-modified for the production of 4-hydroxybutyrate, a precursor of the carbon-four chemical γ-butyrolactone (GBL) (Choi et al., 2013). In fed-batch mode about 6 g L^{-1} of 4-hydroxybutyrate were produced by an engineered strain, which indicates that rumen bacteria are able to produce further carbon-four products beside succinate.

The molecule of interest in this work, β-alanine, is the precursor of 3-hydroxypropionate, a platform chemical (Werpy et al., 2004). Aspartate, the precursor of β-alanine (Leonardi and Jackowski, 2007), is linked to the succinate pathway (**Figure 4.23**).

In *B. succiniciproducens* oxaloacetate is converted to aspartate by an aspartate aminotransferase (*tyrB*, *DD1033*, 1263 bp, 421 amino acids, KEGG database), using glutamate as amino group donor (Fotheringham et al., 1986; Schuster et al., 1999). Additionally, aspartate is connected to the fumarate node by three reactions, comprising first the direct amination by an aspartate ammonia-lyase (*aspA*, *DD0770*, 1398 bp, 466 amino acids, KEGG database). The other two reactions proceed via adenylo-succinate and L-arginino-succinate, which are part of purine metabolism and arginine biosynthesis, respectively (Aimi et al., 1990; Sakanyan et al., 1996; Wang et al., 1995). The product of interest, β-alanine, can be derived from aspartate by an aspartate 1-decarboxylase (*panD*) (Dusch et al., 1999). This enzyme or any other β-alanine producing or consuming enzyme, however, is not found by BLAST search in neither the *M. succiniciproducens* nor the *B. succiniciproducens* genome (KEGG database).

4.4.1 Wild type *Basfia succiniciproducens* does not form β-alanine

When *B. succiniciproducens* DD3, harboring the empty episomal vector pJFF224-XN, was grown in glucose minimal medium supplemented with aspartate (**Figure** *4.22* **A+B**) or β-alanine (**Figure 4.22 C+D**), neither β-alanine formation nor substantial β-alanine consumption was observed. This confirmed the computationally predicted lack of β-alanine formation and consumption in *B. succiniciproducens*.

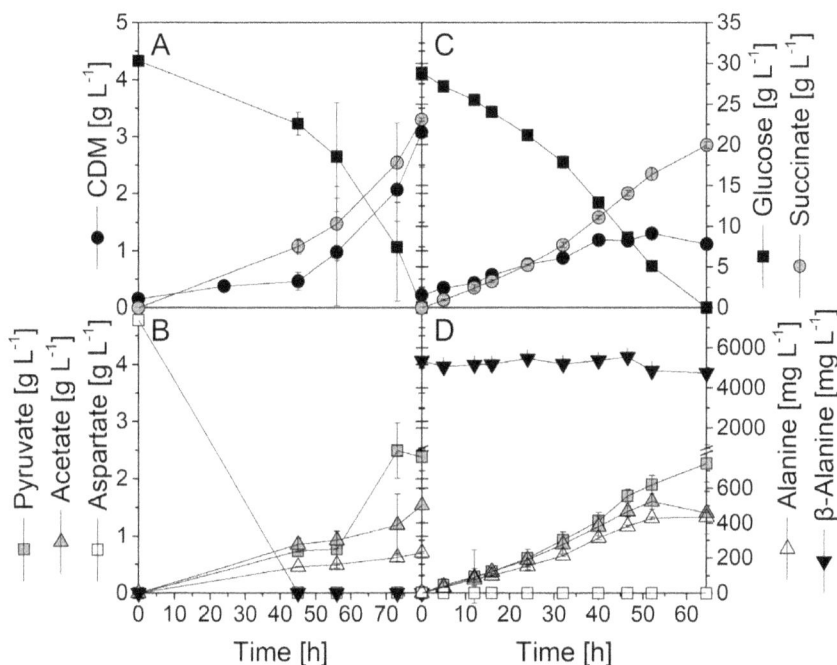

Figure 4.22. Anaerobic growth physiology of *B. succiniciproducens* DD3, harboring the empty vector pJFF224-XN, in serum bottles. To detect β-alanine formation or consumption, cultivation in minimal medium under CO_2 atmosphere was conducted. The constructed strain showed a similar behavior compared to the parent strain. Supplementation of aspartate (**A+B**) enhanced succinate formation, due to anaplerotic fueling of the TCA cycle by conversion of aspartate to oxaloacetate and fumarate. Supplementation with β-alanine (**C+D**) did not affect the performance parameters of the strain. Furthermore no substantial consumption of β-alanine was detectable. Measurement of organic acids, sugars and amino acids was conducted using HPLC. The data represent three independent replicates with means and standard deviations. CDM, Cell dry mass.

4.4.2 Aspartate 1-decarboxylase depicts a possible entry point to β-alanine synthesis

In a previous study, aspartate 1-decarboxylases from *E. coli* and *C. glutamicum* were shown to catalyze the decarboxylation of aspartate into β-alanine, encoded by the *panD* gene (Dusch et al., 1999). To test the suitability of the *E. coli* and *C. glutamicum* *panD* genes for β-alanine synthesis, they were expressed in *B. succiniciproducens*. The "β-alanine production module" was designed in a combinatorial way (**Figure 4.23**). Different promoter-gene combinations, cloned onto the episomal *Pasteurellacea* vector pJFF224-XN (Frey, 1992), were used to identify the most suitable combination.

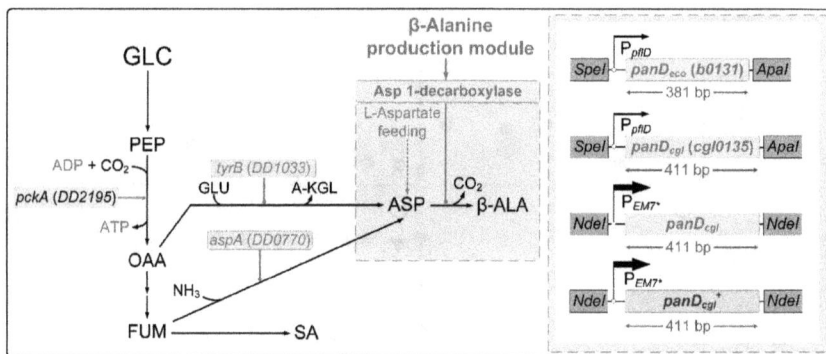

Figure 4.23. Reconstruction of *B. succiniciproducens* DD3 metabolism for β-alanine production. The succinate pathway, specifically aspartate from oxaloacetate and fumarate, was identified as a promising precursor supplier for β-alanine synthesis. A corresponding aspartate 1-decarboxylase, encoded by the gene *panD*, was identified for heterologous β-alanine production, which can be supported by aspartate feeding. Two alternative sources were regarded, *E. coli* and *C. glutamicum*. A codon-optimized version (indicated by a +) of the *panD_cgl* gene was additionally tested. Abbreviations of chemicals are GLC, glucose; PEP, phosphoenolpyruvate; ATP, adenosine triphosphate; ADP, adenosine diphosphate; CO_2, carbon dioxide; OAA, oxaloacetate; FUM, fumarate; NH_3, ammonia; SA, succinic acid; GLU, glutamate; A-KGL, α-ketoglutarate; ASP, aspartate; β-ALA, β-alanine.

4.4.3 Screening for suitable heterologous enzymes for β-alanine synthesis

In the beginning, the identified promoters P_{pflD} and P_{EM7*} were used to implement the β-alanine production module in the strain *B. succiniciproducens* DD3. Thus, cloning of *panD$_{eco}$* and *panD$_{cgl}$* was conducted, yielding the plasmids Bsuc_PL25, Bsuc_PL26 and Bsuc_PL47, respectively (**Figure 6.3**).

The lack of conversion or production of β-alanine in the basic strain *B. succiniciproducens* DD3 + pJFF224-XN, allowed direct screening for suitable *panD* genes, via the resulting β-alanine production from aspartate during anaerobic cultivation (**Figure 4.24**). The cells consumed glucose and aspartate right from the beginning (**Figure 6.4**). The control strain and the strain containing the *panD* gene from *E. coli* did not show substantial β-alanine formation (**Figure 4.24**). In contrast, the use of the *panD$_{cgl}$* gene from *C. glutamicum* enabled the formation of 39 ± 1 mg L^{-1} and 90 ± 3 mg L^{-1} β-alanine when P_{pflD} or P_{EM7*} were used as promoters, respectively. The supplied aspartate was not quantitatively converted to β-alanine. The main fraction of the 5 g L^{-1} of aspartate was channeled into the metabolism elsewhere, most likely into the reductive branch of the TCA cycle, and thus consequently into succinate as shown by the succinic acid titer (**Figure 6.4**).

The use of the obviously stronger *EM7** promoter enabled a 130 % higher β-alanine formation. This P_{EM7*} mediated expression was stronger as compared to that under control of the *pflD* promoter. Still, the β-alanine formed was rather low. To enhance the production, the $(NH_4)_2SO_4$ supplementation was varied, to enforce the *aspA* driven reaction, and to improve the performance of the implemented β-alanine production module.

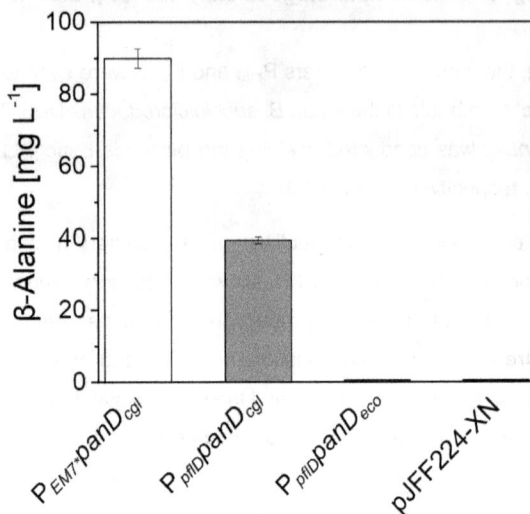

Figure 4.24. Comparison of basic β-alanine producers of *B. succiniciproducens*. To detect β-alanine formation, anaerobic cultivation in glucose minimal medium using aspartate feeding was conducted. After 48 h, the P_{pflD} mediated expression of *panD* from *E. coli* did not show substantial β-alanine production, like the control strain. In contrast, 39 mg L^{-1} was produced using the *panD* gene from *C. glutamicum* under same promoter control. Using the P_{EM7^*} and *panD*$_{cgl}$ enhanced the β-alanine formation up to 89 mg L^{-1}. Measurement of amino acids was conducted using HPLC. The data represent three independent replicates with means and deviation. Cultivation profiles are added to the appendix (**Figure 6.4**).

4.4.4 Determination of the optimal ammonium sulphate concentration

The initial concentration of $(NH_4)_2SO_4$ in the minimal medium was varied, to determine the optimal concentration for β-alanine production. This appeared important, because the precursor aspartate is derived mainly from fumarate, as shown for *E. coli* (Song et al., 2015). The AspA protein uses NH_3 directly for fumarate amination, which is more controllable than the transamination reaction catalyzed by the AspC protein. As a consequence, the intracellular $(NH_4)_2SO_4$ concentration, which is depending on extracellular concentration, plays a role in precursor supply.

The minimal medium contained initial concentrations of 2, 4 and 9 g L^{-1} $(NH_4)_2SO_4$ for cultivation of *B. succiniciproducens* DD3 $P_{EM7}panD_{cgl}$ (**Figure 4.25 A-C**). To study how the different $(NH_4)_2SO_4$ concentrations support the β-alanine formation, the same experiment was conducted with 5 g L^{-1} aspartate (**Figure 4.25 D-F**). Samples were taken after 48 h and processed by HPLC analysis. This revealed that β-alanine formation was possible without supplementing aspartate, whereby the $(NH_4)_2SO_4$ amount had an impact on the β-alanine formation. The maximum production (62 ± 1 mg L^{-1}) was detected, using 4 g L^{-1} of supplemented ammonium (**Figure 4.25 B**). When 2 g L^{-1} (**Figure 4.25 A**) or 9 g L^{-1} (**Figure 4.25 C**) of $(NH_4)_2SO_4$ were supplemented, 35 ± 9.0 mg L^{-1} and 41 ± 0 mg L^{-1} of β-alanine were formed, respectively.

A maximum β-alanine titer of 100 ± 1 mg L^{-1} was reached when aspartate was supplemented, accompanied by use of 4 g L^{-1} $(NH_4)_2SO_4$. When 2 g L^{-1} $(NH_4)_2SO_4$ was supplied, the β-alanine titer decreased slightly. In contrast, the highest $(NH_4)_2SO_4$ concentration (9 g L^{-1}) caused a decrease of the β-alanine titer (50.3 ± 0.9 mg L^{-1} β-alanine).

The highest ammonium supplementation decreased growth substantially, either without or with aspartate supplementation. This seemed one reason for the lowered β-alanine production under these conditions. To implement these results in further β-alanine production experiments, 4 g L^{-1} of $(NH_4)_2SO_4$ were added.

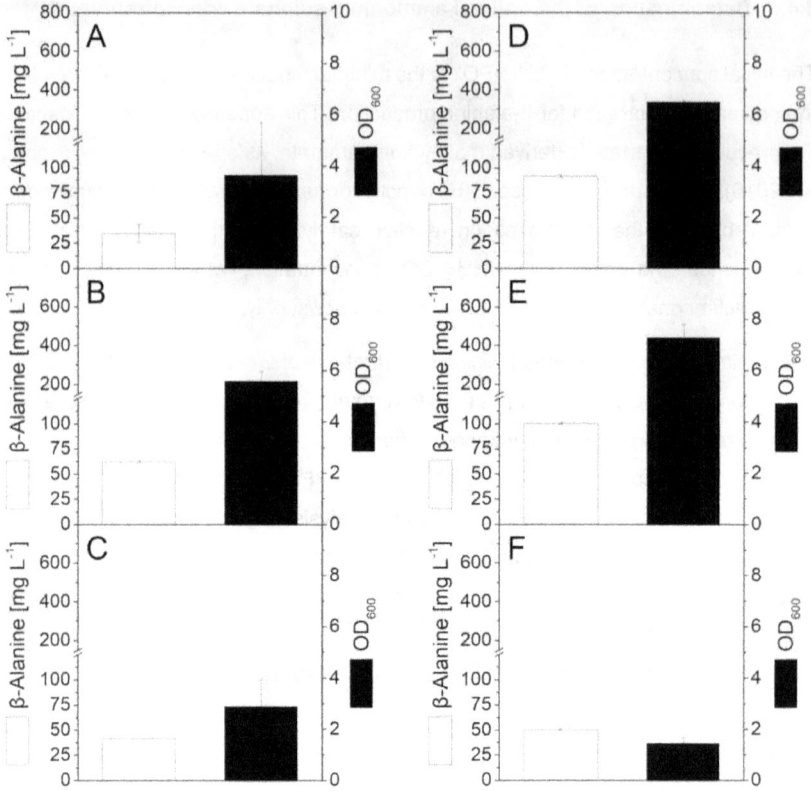

Figure 4.25. Influence of varied (NH₄)₂SO₄ supplementation on β-alanine formation using *B. succiniciproducens* DD3 + P*EM7*-panD*cgl*. The strain was anaerobically grown in minimal medium for 48 h before sampling. Different concentrations of $(NH_4)_2SO_4$ (2 g L^{-1}: **A+D**; 4 g L^{-1}: **B+E**; 9 g L^{-1}: **C+F**) were used. For comparison, the minimal medium was used lean (**A, B, C**) or with supplementation of 5 g L^{-1} aspartate (**D, E, F**). Measurement of β-alanine was conducted using HPLC. The data represent duplicates with means and deviation

4.4.5 Codon optimization of the *panD* gene

To increase and stabilize the expression of the *panD* gene from *C. glutamicum*, and consequently the corresponding enzyme activity, a codon-optimized version was synthesized (**Sequence 6.1**). The codon-optimized *panD$_{cgl}$+* gene was cloned onto the pJFF224-XN vector under control of the *pflD* or the *EM7** promoter, yielding Bsuc_PL80 (P$_{EM7}$·*panD$_{cgl}$+)* and Bsuc_PL86 (P$_{pflD}$*panD$_{cgl}$+*) (**Figure 6.5**).

Minimal medium cultivation of the constructed strains was conducted (**Figure 4.26**). As before, 5 g L^{-1} aspartate was either supplemented (**Figure 4.26 A-C, G-I**) or omitted (**Figure 4.26 D-F, J-L**) from the medium. The strains revealed a similar physiology as before. Glucose was consumed from early on. The strain DD3 P$_{pflD}$*panD$_{cgl}$+* produced 42.5 ± 0.0 mg L^{-1} β-alanine without aspartate and 38 ± 0.0 mg L^{-1} with aspartate supplementation. Increased production of about 105.3 ± 4.9 mg L^{-1} β-alanine was observed for DD3 P$_{EM7}$·*panD$_{cgl}$+*, which was even improved further (187.6 ± 10.2 mg L^{-1}), when aspartate was supplemented. The strains grew up to a biomass concentration of about 2 g$_{CDM}$ L^{-1} and 3.5 g$_{CDM}$ L^{-1} without and with aspartate supplementation, respectively. The biomass formation was clearly enhanced, when aspartate was supplied. Aspartate supplementation again enhanced succinate formation. Here, an increase from 19.9 ± 0.2 g L^{-1} (**Figure 4.26 B+H**) to 23.4 ± 0.2 g L^{-1} succinate (**Figure 4.26 E+K**) was observable.

Regarding β-alanine production, the *EM7** promoter was found superior, as observed before. Coupling the strong *EM7** promoter and the optimal codon usage of the *panD$_{cgl}$* gene, the β-alanine production was improved by 163 %, as compared to the first generation producer strain DD3 P$_{pflD}$*panD$_{cgl}$*. When the direct precursor aspartate was supplied, the production was even enhanced by 369 %.

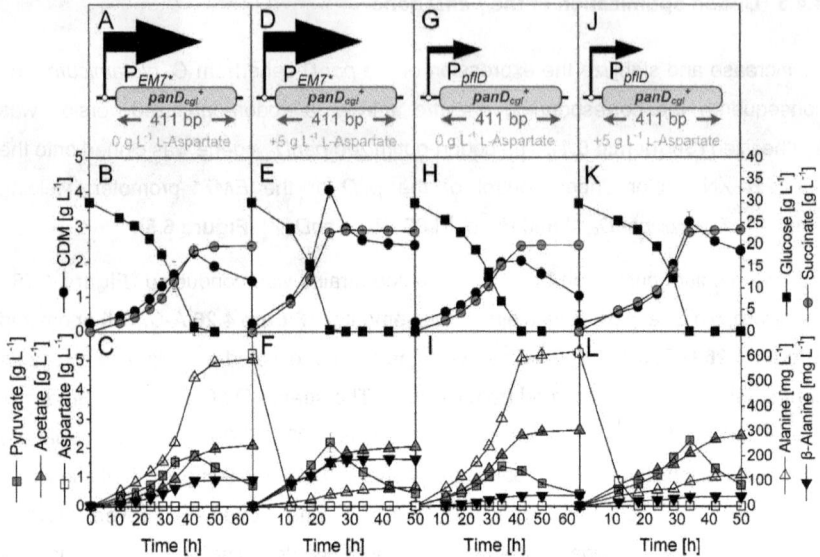

Figure 4.26. Comparison of anaerobic growth physiology of second generation β-alanine producer strains of *B. succiniciproducens* DD3. The strains *B. succiniciproducens* DD3 + $P_{pflD}panD_{cgl}^+$ (A-C, D-F) and DD3 $P_{EM7^*}·panD_{cgl}^+$ (G-I, J-L) contain a codon-optimized version (indicated by the +) of the $panD_{cgl}$ gene. A subsequent cultivation under anaerobic (CO_2) conditions in glucose minimal medium was conducted. For comparison, medium was used lean (A, G) or supplemented with 5 g L⁻¹ aspartate (D, J). Native succinate production (B, H) was found to be improved by aspartate supplementation (E, K) confirming a drain of aspartate carbon into succinate. Although, no substantial increase in β-alanine production was detected (42.5 mg L⁻¹ in 42 h), when *pflD* promoter was used, either with aspartate. An improvement to 105 mg L⁻¹ of β-alanine was reached, when the *EM7** promoter was deployed in combination with the codon-optimized $panD_{cgl}^+$ gene. A further improvement of about 78 % (187 mg L⁻¹) was achieved, when the latter was supplied with aspartate. Measurement of organic acids, sugars and amino acids was conducted using HPLC. The data represent three independent replicates with means and standard deviations. CDM, Cell dry mass.

4.4.6 Harnessing the *panP* gene from *Vibrio natriegens* for β-alanine production

Due to the low titers, the used *panD* genes appeared non-optimal for β-alanine production in *B. succiniciproducens*. Commonly, β-alanine is synthesized by similar pyruvoyl-dependent PanD proteins, which are found in many organisms, e.g. *E. coli* and *C. glutamicum* (Dusch et al., 1999; Stuecker et al., 2012). This enzyme is expressed as an inactive pro-protein and is then cleaved to yield the active protein (Stuecker et al., 2012). This mechanism, however, might have been not properly functioning in *B. succiniciproducens*.

Recent work (Pan et al., 2017) uncovered, that another protein family, namely PanP, provides also aspartate 1-decarboxylase activity, but is suggested to be pyridoxal-dependent. The PanP proteins are commonly found in a number of marine bacteria, including *Vibrio fischeri* (Pan et al., 2017). The lately evoked interest in the marine bacterium *V. natriegens* (Fernández-Llamosas et al., 2017; Hoffart et al., 2017; Lee et al., 2016; Long et al., 2017; Maida et al., 2013; Weinstock et al., 2016) was a trigger to search for such a *panP* gene in this microbe.

A BLAST search on the protein level, using the *V. fischeri* PanP protein (glutamate decarboxylase, EC 4.1.1.15, KEGG entry: VF0892) against the *V. natriegens* genome was conducted. This identified a homologous protein (86 %), annotated as a glutamate decarboxylase (glutamate decarboxylase, EC 4.1.1.15, KEGG entry: PN96_07390). On DNA level, 72 % similarity was found. This protein (548 amino acids) is longer than the PanD protein (136 amino acids). This implicates different properties or even reaction mechanisms, which could be more suitable for β-alanine synthesis in *B. succiniciproducens* than the examined PanD proteins. No evidence of such a PanP related protein in *B. succiniciproducens* was found by BLAST search.

It was not known if this protein produces β-alanine from aspartate. The gene PN96_07390 was cloned onto pJFF224-XN under P_{EM7}. control, yielding Bsuc_PL105 (**Figure 6.6**). Subsequent cultivation of the cloning host *E. coli* DH10B in minimal medium, revealed substantial *De-novo* production of β-alanine, as compared to the control strain, containing only the empty vector pJFF224-XN (**Figure 6.7**).

After subsequent construction of the corresponding *B. succiniproducens* strain (**Figure 6.6**), a minimal medium cultivation either without or with 5 g L^{-1} aspartate supplementation was conducted (**Figure 4.27**). Deploying the *panP* gene enabled significant β-alanine formation in *B. succiniciproducens*. The titer increased to

161 ± 11 mg L^{-1} without aspartate supplementation (**Figure 4.27 A+B**). When aspartate was added, even 446 ± 31 mg L^{-1} β-alanine was formed, but cell growth was somehow impaired (**Figure 4.27 C+D**). Additionally, the depletion of the supplied aspartate, was accompanied by a decreased β-alanine production rate. While aspartate was available, a volumetric productivity of 26.7 mg β-alanine L^{-1} h^{-1} was observed. After the aspartate was consumed, this value decreased to 2.8 mg L^{-1} h^{-1}, almost similar compared to the cultivation without aspartate (6.5 mg L^{-1} h^{-1}). This indicated that aspartate supply is a bottleneck in the synthesis of β-alanine in *B. succiniciproducens*, independently of the used aspartate 1-decarboxylase.

Taken together, use of the novel *panP* gene enabled highest β-alanine production performance compared to the best second generation strain, which contained the *panD*$_{cgl}$$^+$ gene. Future codon optimization of the *V. natriegens* *panP* might further improve the performance.

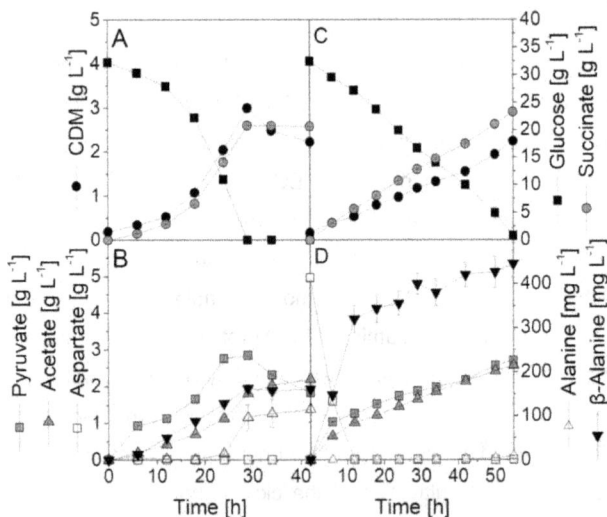

Figure 4.27. Growth physiology of a *B. succiniciproducens* DD3 strain containing the *panP*$_{vna}$ gene from *V. natriegens* under P$_{EM7}$ control. Glucose minimal medium was used either lean or with 5 g L^{-1} of aspartate supplementation. An increased β-alanine production was observed in lean medium (160 mg L^{-1}). The latter was improved by aspartate supplementation to about 450 mg L^{-1}. Organic acids, sugars and amino acids were measured using HPLC. The data represent three independent replicates with means and deviation. CDM, Cell dry mass.

Next, enzyme assays for the implemented PanD aspartate 1-decarboxylases were conducted (**Table 6.3**). In short, the negative control showed no formation of β-alanine and no aspartate consumption, respectively (**Figure 4.28 A**). The control strain revealed no β-alanine formation, but consumption of aspartate (10.8 mg L^{-1} h^{-1}) (**Figure 4.28 B**). The crude extract, containing the native PanD$_{cgl}$ enzyme, showed a β-alanine formation rate of 4.5 ± 0.3 mg L^{-1} h^{-1}, corresponding to a specific activity of 4.6 ± 0.3 mU mg$_{protein}^{-1}$ (**Figure 4.28 C + F**). The aspartate consumption was increased (16.8 mg L^{-1} h^{-1}) compared to the control, due to the additional aspartate depletion by PanD$_{cgl}$. An increased β-alanine formation (7.4 ± 0.6 mg L^{-1} h^{-1}) (**Figure 4.28 D**) was observed, using the codon-optimized *panD$_{cgl}$*⁺ gene, corresponding to a specific activity of 7.3 mU mg^{-1} (**Figure 4.28 F**). Obviously, the codon optimization improved gene expression, and consequently the specific activity of PanD$_{cgl}$ by 59 %. PanP showed a loss of activity after 1 h of incubation. A substantial lower specific activity of 1.2 ± 0.6 mU mg^{-1} was derived from the data, although this enzyme was shown to yield better producer strains than the PanD$_{cgl}$ enzyme. It was assumed, that the used assay conditions were not suitable for this type of enzyme, due to a lack of pyridoxal 5-phosphate. Therefore, supplementation of pyridoxal 5-phosphate and selected assay conditions (Pan et al., 2017) were tested in an additional PanP enzyme assay.

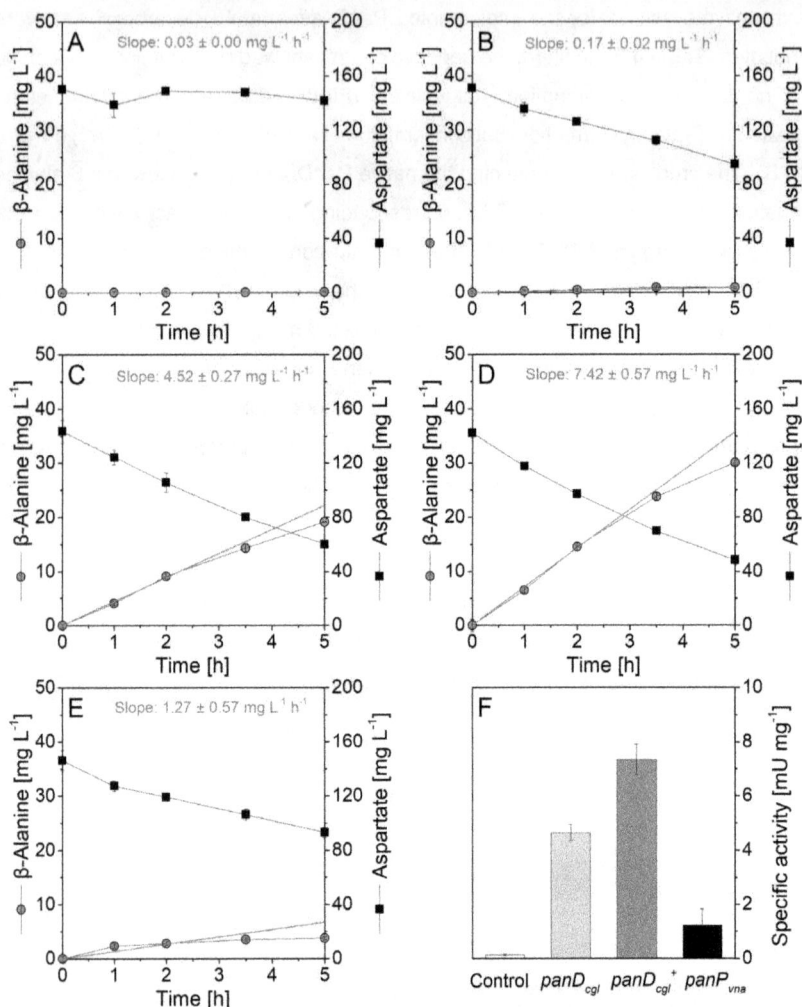

Figure 4.28. Results of the PanD aspartate 1-decarboxylase assay. Crude extracts of *B. succiniciproducens* DD3 + P*EM7*panD*cgl*, DD3 + P*EM7*panD*cgl*+, DD3 + P*EM7*panP*vna* and the control strain, containing pJFF224-XN, were used for the aspartate 1-decarboxlase assay. The water control (**A**) showed no significant aspartate consumption or β-alanine formation. The control extract converted aspartate but no β-alanine formation was observable (**B**). Distinct β-alanine formation rates were obtained for the crude extracts of DD3 + P*EM7*panD*cgl* (**C**), DD3 + P*EM7*panD*cgl*+ (**D**) and DD3 + P*EM7*panP*vna* (**E**). The obtained β-alanine formation rates were converted to specific enzyme activities, using the measured protein concentration of the crude extracts (**F**). Amino acids were measured using HPLC. The data represent three independent replicates with means and standard deviations.

Similarly, to the PanD assay, the negative control of the PanP assay showed neither β-alanine formation nor aspartate consumption (**Figure 4.29 A**). The control strain extract formed no β-alanine, but elevated aspartate consumption was observed in the first hour (up to 300 mg L^{-1} h^{-1}) (**Figure 4.29 B**). The crude extract, which expressed the codon-optimized $panD_{cgl}^+$ showed a similar specific activity of 10.15 ± 0.17 mU mg^{-1}, when compared to the PanD assay. This corresponded to an increase in aspartate consumption (357 mg L^{-1}) (**Figure 4.29 C**). Obviously, the highest activity showed the $PanP_{vna}$ enzyme (**Figure 4.29 D**). The specific activity (264 mU mg^{-1}) was superior compared to $PanD_{cgl}$. Consequently, the aspartate consumption was furthermore increased (665 mg L^{-1} h^{-1}). In regard of the decreasing enzyme activity during the assay, it was decided to test $PanP_{vna}$ once again under these conditions. Samples were taken during the first hour of the assay, which allowed determination of the enzyme's maximum specific activity (**Figure 4.29 E**). A maximum β-alanine formation rate of up to 445 mg L^{-1} h^{-1} was measured. The corresponding maximum specific activity of the enzyme was 372.66 ± 19.61 mU mg^{-1}.

The enzyme assay confirmed the observed advantages of $PanP_{vna}$ in *B. succiniciproducens*. A 37-fold improvement of the specific activity was reached, compared to the codon-optimized expressed $PanD_{cgl}$ enzyme. It is concluded that the $PanP_{vna}$ reaction mechanism, relying on pyridoxal 5-phosphate, is advantageous compared to the $PanD_{cgl}$ protein. It is assumed, that a major hurdle regarding the low activity of the $PanD_{cgl}$ enzyme, may its cleavage mechanism to yield the active protein, which is not fully functional in *B. succiniciproducens*.

As shown for the $panD_{cgl}$ gene, a codon-optimization of the $panP_{vna}$ gene can additionally improve β-alanine production. Furthermore, the crude extracts of *B. succiniciproducens* showed a conversion of aspartate *in vitro* to, so far, unknown metabolites. A competition between β-alanine forming and aspartate consuming enzymes is the consequence. This depicts a target for future metabolic engineering to improve aspartate supply and diminish competitive aspartate consuming reactions.

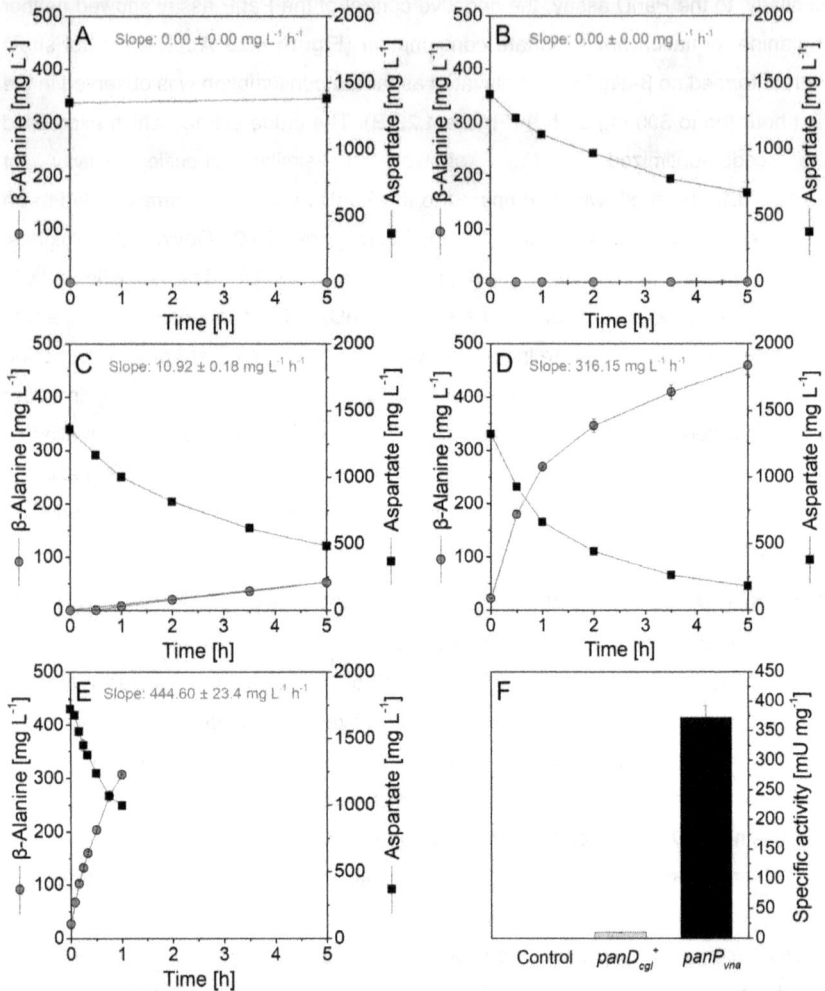

Figure 4.29. Results of the PanP aspartate 1-decarboxylase assay. Crude extracts of *B. succiniciproducens* DD3 + P_{EM7}-$panD_{cgl}^+$, DD3 + P_{EMT}-$panP_{vna}$ and the control strain, containing pJFF224-XN, were used. No significant aspartate consumption or β-alanine formation was shown by the water control (**A**). The control extract converted aspartate but no β-alanine formation was observed (**B**). A similar β-alanine formation rate compared to the PanD assay was obtained using the crude extract of DD3 + P_{EMT}-$panD_{cgl}$ (**C**). The crude extract of DD3 + P_{EMT}-$panP_{vna}$ showed the highest β-alanine formation rate during this study (**D, E**). The obtained β-alanine formation rates were converted to specific enzyme activities, using the measured protein concentration of the crude extracts (**F**). Amino acids were measured using HPLC. The data represent three independent replicates with means and standard deviations.

4.5 Metabolic engineering for 3-hydroxypropionate production

The achieved β-alanine production now opened the possibility to derive 3-HP via the β-alanine route. This pathway appeared promising, due to its negative ΔG^0 (-32.3 kJ mol^{-1}) (Valdehuesa et al., 2013).

4.5.1 Conversion of β-alanine to 3-hydroxypropionate – concept and plasmid construction

A closer look at the pathway (**Figure 4.30 A**) revealed that NADP$^+$ is supplied for NADPH regeneration. In addition pyruvate is needed in the β-alanine transamination step to malonate semialdehyde and alanine.

It comprised two more enzymes. One enzyme: a β-alanine pyruvate transaminase, catalyzing the amino group transfer from β-alanine to pyruvate, yielding malonate semialdehyde and alanine (Ingram et al., 2007), and a malonate semialdehyde reductase to reduce malonate semialdehyde by use of NADPH (Fujisawa et al., 2003). There was no evidence of a β-alanine pyruvate transaminase present in the genome of *B. succiniciproducens*. Hence, it was decided to use a heterologous gene (*bapta$_{ppu}$*) from *P. putida* KT2440 (beta-alanine--pyruvate transaminase, EC 2.6.1.18, PP_0596, KEGG database). Blast search of a malonate semialdehyde reductase against the *B. succiniciproducens* genome, i.e. *ydfG* from *E. coli* K12 MG1655, identified the *dltE* gene as a similar homologue on protein level (61 % identities). Due to the unknown function of the *dltE* gene, it was decided to use the heterologous *ydfG* (*ydfG$_{eco}$*) gene from *E. coli* K12 MG1655.

Both genes were synthesized, with regard to the *B. succiniciproducens* codon-usage (indicated by a $^+$), in a polycistronic design under *pflD* promoter control (**Figure 4.30 B 1.)**). The gene combination was designated as the "3-HP production module" (plasmid Bsuc_PL27). In a next step, the synthesis of 3-HP from glucose was tested. Therefore two operons comprising the genes *panD$_{cgl}$* / *panDcgl$^+$*, *bapta$_{ppu}$$^+$* and *ydfG$_{eco}$$^+$*, were designed (**Figure 4.30 B 2.) + 3.)**). This organized *panD$_{cgl}$* or *panDcgl$^+$*, *bapta$_{ppu}$$^+$*, and *ydfG$_{eco}$$^+$* under control of the strong *EM7** promoter. For translation, the P$_{EM7^*}$ ribosomal binding site (*RBS$_{EM7^*}$*, 18 bp), was implemented between *panD$_{cgl}$* / *panDcgl$^+$*, *bapta$_{ppu}$* and *ydfG$_{eco}$*, respectively.

The two designs were realized by cloning the individual fragments onto the episomal vector pJFF224-XN by use of Gibson's Assembly (**Figure 4.30 B**) (**Figure 6.8**). The derived plasmids were named Bsuc_PL52, and Bsuc_PL98 (**Table 2.1**).

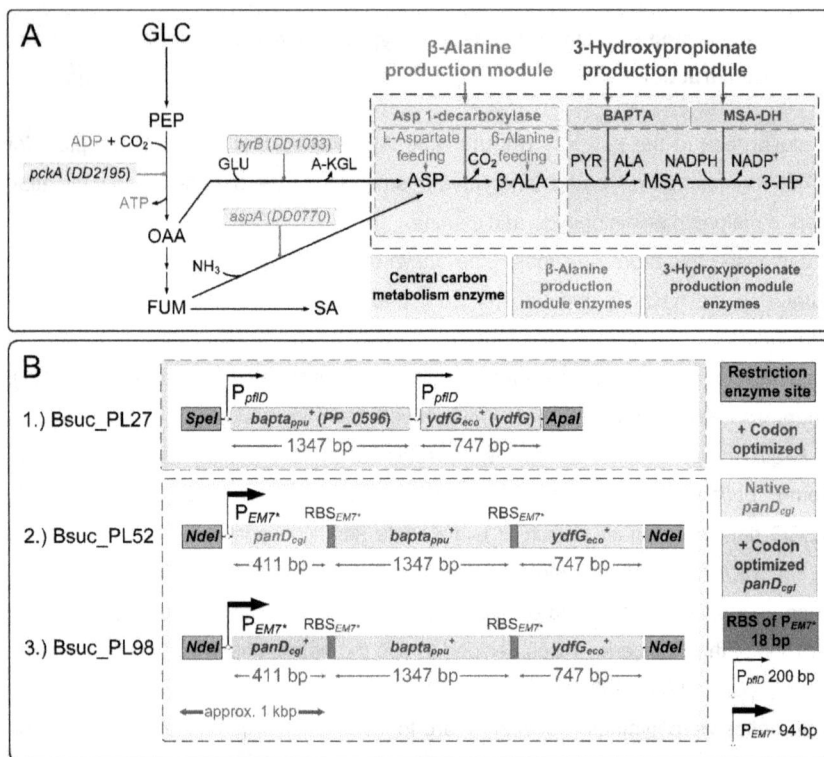

Figure 4.30. Reconstruction of *B. succiniciproducens* DD3 metabolism for 3-HP production. The β-alanine synthesis pathway was enhanced by use of the 3-HP production module (**A**). *P. putida* KT2440 and *E. coli* K12 MG1655 were chosen as sources for the genes *bapta_{ppu}^+* and *ydfG_{eco}^+*, respectively. Different constructs (**B**) for heterologous gene expression allowing 3-HP production from β-alanine or glucose were cloned onto pJFF224-XN. Abbreviations of chemicals are GLC, glucose; PEP, phosphoenolpyruvate; ATP, adenosine triphosphate; ADP, adenosine diphosphate; CO_2, carbon dioxide; OAA, oxaloacetate; FUM, fumarate; NH_3, ammonia; SA, succinic acid; GLU, glutamate; A-KGL, α-ketoglutarate; ASP, aspartate; β-ALA, β-alanine; PYR, pyruvate; ALA, alanine; MSA, malonate semialdehyde; NADPH, nicotineamide adenine dinucleotide phosphate, reduced; $NADP^+$, nicotineamide adenine dinucleotide phosphate, oxidized; 3-HP, 3-hydroxypropionate.

4.5.2 There is no native 3-hydroxypropionate metabolism in *Basfia succiniciproducens*

To test if the cells were able to consume 3-HP, a minimal medium cultivation with 5 g L^{-1} supplemented 3-HP was conducted using *B. succiniciproducens* DD3 + pJFF224-XN (**Figure 4.31**). After a substantial lag phase (**Figure 6.9**), the cells grew up to 48 h until the initial glucose amount was consumed. The succinate yield was rather unaffected. Although, the *dltE* gene of *B. succiniciproducens* is potentially related to 3-HP conversion, 3-HP consumption was not observed (**Figure 4.31**, **Figure 6.10**). This experiment suggested the feasibility of converting glucose to β-alanine and consequently to 3-HP by *B. succiniciproducens*, without undesired conversion of the final product.

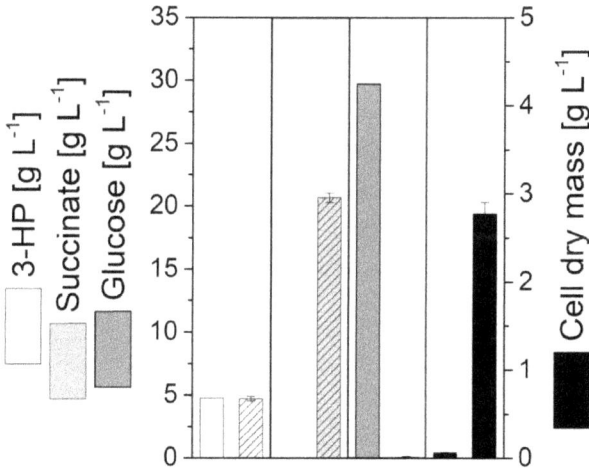

Figure 4.31. Influence of 3-HP on the anaerobic growth physiology of *B. succiniciproducens* DD3 + pJFF224-XN in serum bottles. To detect conversion of 3-HP (white bars), 5 g L^{-1} were supplemented in glucose (dark grey bars) minimal medium. Cell growth (black bars) was normally after a substantial lag phase of 36 h. The 0 h (open bars) and the 48 h (hatched bars) samples were processed via HPLC. There is no evidence of 3-HP conversion by the used strain. Succinate (light grey bars) production was not impaired by 3-HP supplementation.

4.5.3 The 3-hydroxypropionate production module is functional in *Basfia succiniciproducens*

The plasmid Bsuc_PL27, containing the 3-HP production module, was successfully transformed into *B. succiniciproducens* DD3. Subsequently, a cultivation under anaerobic conditions (CO_2) was conducted in minimal medium. To prove the functionality of the 3-HP production module, 5 g L^{-1} β-alanine was added (**Figure 4.32 A-C**). In addition, a control experiment omitting β-alanine supplementation was conducted (**Figure 4.32 D-F**).

3-HP production occurred, when β-alanine was supplemented, whereas no production occurred without supplementation. After 72 h, 217 ± 4 mg L^{-1} 3-HP was produced. The presence of 3-HP in the supernatant was verified via GC-MS (**Figure 6.11**). Surprisingly, β-alanine was not converted in an equimolar ratio. The initial β-alanine concentration of 5 g L^{-1} was reduced by 813 ± 39 mg L^{-1}. Thus, 596 mg L^{-1} of the consumed β-alanine were not recovered in the product: 73 % of the β-alanine carbon fraction was used in an unknown manner. In comparison to the parent strain, and non-producing condition, significant alanine production was observed. This confirmed that the Bapta$_{ppu}$ enzyme used pyruvate as co-factor (Song et al., 2016).

To sum it up, the 3-HP production module was found active and functional in *B. succiniciproducens* and converted β-alanine to 3-HP. Furthermore, an unknown conversion of β-alanine was observed. In the next step, β-alanine and 3-HP production modules were combined to produce 3-HP from glucose.

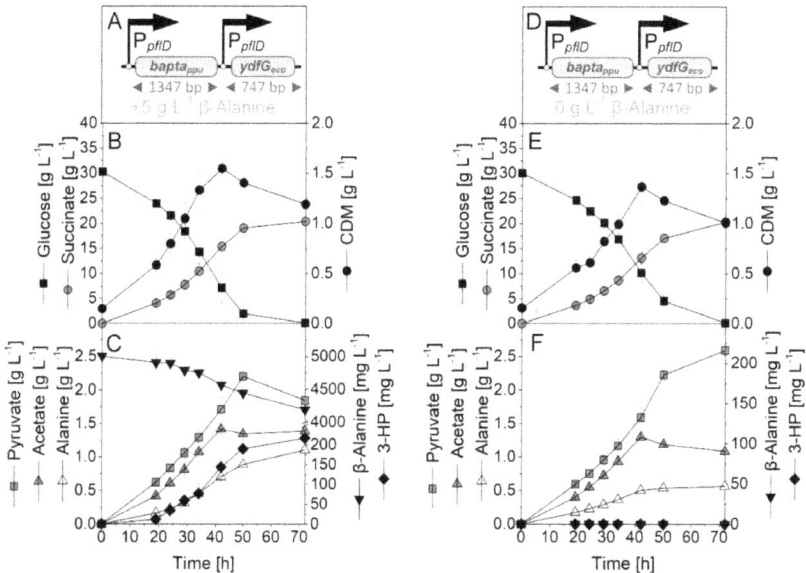

Figure 4.32. Anaerobic growth physiology of a first generation 3-HP producer strain of B. succiniciproducens DD3. The strain B. succiniciproducens DD3 $P_{pflD}bapta_{ppu}^+$-$P_{pflD}ydfG_{eco}^+$ contains a codon-optimized version (indicated by the +) of the 3-HP production module genes. A glucose minimal medium cultivation under anaerobic (CO_2) conditions was conducted. For comparison, medium was supplemented with 5 g L^{-1} β-alanine (**A**) or used lean (**D**). Native succinate production (**B, E**) was found. When β-alanine was supplied (**C**), a substantial production of 3-HP (217 mg L^{-1}) was observed. Without supplemented β-alanine (**F**), no 3-HP formation was found. Measurement of organic acids, sugars and amino acids was conducted using HPLC. The data represent three independent replicates with means and standard deviations. CDM, Cell dry mass.

4.5.4 Combination of the β-alanine and 3-HP production module

The cloned plasmid Bsuc_PL52 represented an operon of the genes $panD_{cgl}$, $bapta_{ppu}^+$ and $ydfG_{eco}^+$ with the strong *EM7** promoter as control element. After successful transformation into *B. succiniciproducens* DD3, a glucose minimal medium cultivation under anaerobic (CO_2) conditions was conducted (**Figure 4.33 A+B**). To determine the influence of the single precursor metabolites in the pathway, aspartate (**Figure 4.33 C+D**) or β-alanine (**Figure 4.33 E+F**) were supplemented at an initial concentration of 5 g L^{-1} each.

The strain consumed glucose and native succinate production was observed (**Figure 4.33 A**). When neither aspartate nor β-alanine were supplemented, only minor 3-HP amounts were detected (**Figure 4.33 B**), hard to distinguish from background noise of the HPLC chromatogram. Aspartate supplementation (**Figure 4.33 C**) enhanced succinate production and cell growth and stimulated 3-HP production (**Figure 4.33 D**) (46 ± 1 mg L^{-1}). Supplementation of β-alanine had no effect on succinate production and cell growth (**Figure 4.33 E**), but increased 3-HP production to 569 ± 13 mg L^{-1} (**Figure 4.33 F**). This was an improvement by 160 %, as compared to the initial experiment. Furthermore, 3-HP overproduction was accompanied by alanine formation (up to 2.2 ± 0.0 g L^{-1}).

Obviously, the PanD$_{cgl}$ enzyme displayed a bottleneck in the synthetic pathway. This indicated that the PanD$_{cgl}$ protein was not sufficiently expressed or active. A lack of the *panD$_{cgl}$* gene expression is unlikely, due to the polycistronic expression design, which enabled significant β-alanine consumption and 3-HP production by the Bapta$_{ppu}$ and the YdfG$_{eco}$ enzyme. Unknown issues, regarding maturing and folding impair the enzyme activity of the PanD$_{cgl}$ protein in the *B. succiniciproducens* cytosol, which results in a slow conversion of aspartate to β-alanine.

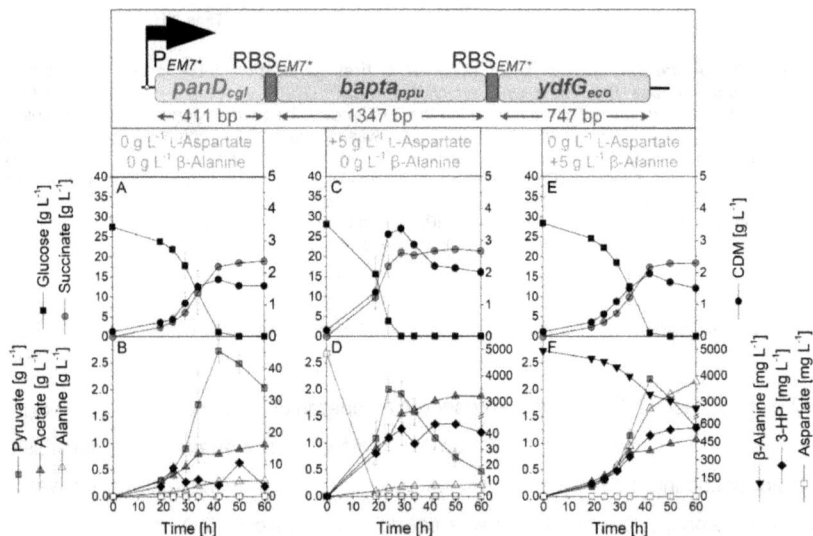

Figure 4.33. Anaerobic growth physiology of a second generation 3-HP producer strain of *B. succiniciproducens* DD3. The strain *B. succiniciproducens* DD3 P$_{EM7*}$panD$_{cgl}$-RBS$_{EM7*}$-bapta$_{ppu}$+-RBS$_{EM7*}$-ydfG$_{eco}$+ contains all 3-HP production genes under *EM7** promoter control. A glucose minimal medium cultivation under anaerobic (CO$_2$) conditions was conducted. When the medium was used lean, the native succinate production (**A**) was found and only minor 3-HP traces were produced (**B**). When aspartate was supplied, succinate production was raised as observed before (**C**). Additionally, a small but significant 3-HP production (46 mg L^{-1}) was observed (**D**). Supplementation of β-alanine had no significant influence on succinate production (**E**), but enabled a substantial 3-HP formation (569 mg L^{-1}) (**F**). Measurement of organic acids, sugars and amino acids was conducted using HPLC. The data represent three independent replicates with means and standard deviations. CDM, Cell dry mass.

The 3-HP operon was proven to be functional, upon regulation by a single promoter. The synthetic, non-natural transcription unit indicated, that transcription and translation was promoted by the *EM7** promoter and the RBS_{EM7^*} binding site, respectively.

4.5.5 Characteristics of the β-alanine carbon loss in the 3-HP production strain

To study the undesired loss of β-alanine carbon, labeled $[^{13}C\text{-}^{15}N]$-β-alanine was used in a feeding experiment with *B. succiniciproducens* DD3 + Bsuc_PL52. This should additionally verify the transamination reaction of pyruvate to alanine by the Bapta$_{ppu}$ enzyme.

The strain grew as before (**Figure 4.33 E+F**). After glucose was consumed, biomass and supernatant samples were taken for measuring mass isotope distributions of selected organic acids and amino acids (**Figure 4.34**). The mass distributions were corrected for naturally occurring isotopes (van Winden et al., 2002). The obtained data are given in **Table 6.4** and **Table 6.5**.

The 3-HP production via the β-alanine route was shown to be accompanied by accumulation of alanine. This is a result of the β-alanine conversion to malonate semialdehyde via the transamination of pyruvate to alanine. This was shown by the m+1 mass shift of the detected alanine fragment (**Figure 4.34 A**), resulting from the ^{15}N incorporation of the deployed β-alanine. The formed alanine was not recovered by the production strain, hence a loss of carbon into alanine is the consequence. This phenomenon was not yet described in other studies using the β-alanine route (Borodina et al., 2015; Song et al., 2016). It is thought, that the lack of alanine recovery is a distinct property of *B. succiniciproducens, which* impairs the 3-HP production negatively. This phenomenon may not be present in other used microorganisms.

Furthermore, it could be proven that the 3-HP carbon skeleton originated from β-alanine, due to the detected m+3 labeling (**Figure 4.34 B**).

The fact that neither β-alanine nor 3-HP was converted by the parent strain, suggests that carbon from β-alanine must be re-routed at the level of malonate semialdehyde (**Figure 4.34 C**). Unknown enzyme reactions using this compound had to be considered. Genome analysis (KEGG database) of the related genus *Mannheimia* showed presence of a gene, which may cause methylmalonate-semialdehyde dehydrogenase (EC 1.2.1.18) activity. This enzyme is predicted to form acetyl-CoA from malonate semialdehyde, using oxidative decarboxylation (KEGG database) (Hayaishi et al., 1961). The enzyme is annotated in *M. haemolytica* and *M. variegena*.

When a protein BLAST of the corresponding proteins was conducted against the *B. succiniciproducens* proteom, a protein (PutA, *DD1522*) with a similarity of about 29 %, and positive matching residues of 47 % was found. This gene and the corresponding enzyme activity is thought to cause the observed loss of β-alanine carbon. The corresponding protein showed aldehyde dehydrogenase motifs, but interestingly differed in a great extent when compared to another annotated aldehyde dehydrogenase (PutA, *DD2045*).

To study the potential acetyl-CoA formation from β-alanine, labeling in the acetyl-CoA pool and related pools was considered. If labeled carbon from the β-alanine pool was converted into acetyl-CoA, subsequent ^{13}C enrichment of acetate, glutamate and accordingly, proline should result. Exactly this was found (**Figure 4.34 D-F**). The most significant signature of the ^{13}C-β-alanine carbon was found in the C_2 compound acetate, which is derived from acetyl-CoA. Accordingly, a m+2 mass shift was observed here, indicating labeled carbon, originating from acetyl-CoA and thus from β-alanine. Additionally, the carbon backbone of glutamate and proline showed the m+2 mass shift. These results indicated that carbon from ^{13}C-^{15}N-β-alanine was recovered here, which is then consequently channeled into biomass. But other biomass compounds did not show significant ^{13}C enrichments. A few amino acids possessed a small m+1 labeling originating more likely from the ^{15}N from β-alanine, distributed in the metabolism.

One reasonable explanation of the missing biomass compound labeling is its distribution from acetyl-CoA to malonyl-CoA into fatty acids. This has to be considered carefully, due to the *pflD* knockout in the parent strain. Thus, 16 % of the flux from pyruvate to formate, and consequently into acetyl-CoA is withdrawn (Becker et al., 2013). Hence, the latter may accentuate a substantial shortage of acetyl-CoA, yielding a lack of fatty acid precursors. Measuring the labeling in the fatty acid fraction of the biomass may unravel the missing labeling of the β-alanine carbon in future studies.

It was shown, that β-alanine is converted into malonate semialdehyde, which is withdrawn from the synthetic 3-HP pathway into acetyl-CoA. Acetyl-CoA is then converted into compounds of the biomass. This carbon loss, the alanine formation in the pathway, and the missing alanine recovery reduces the 3-HP synthesis performance by 73 %. It is concluded, that a knockout of the gene *putA* (*DD1522*) and implementation of alanine recovering enzymes may improve the performance of the *B. succiniciproducens* 3-HP producer.

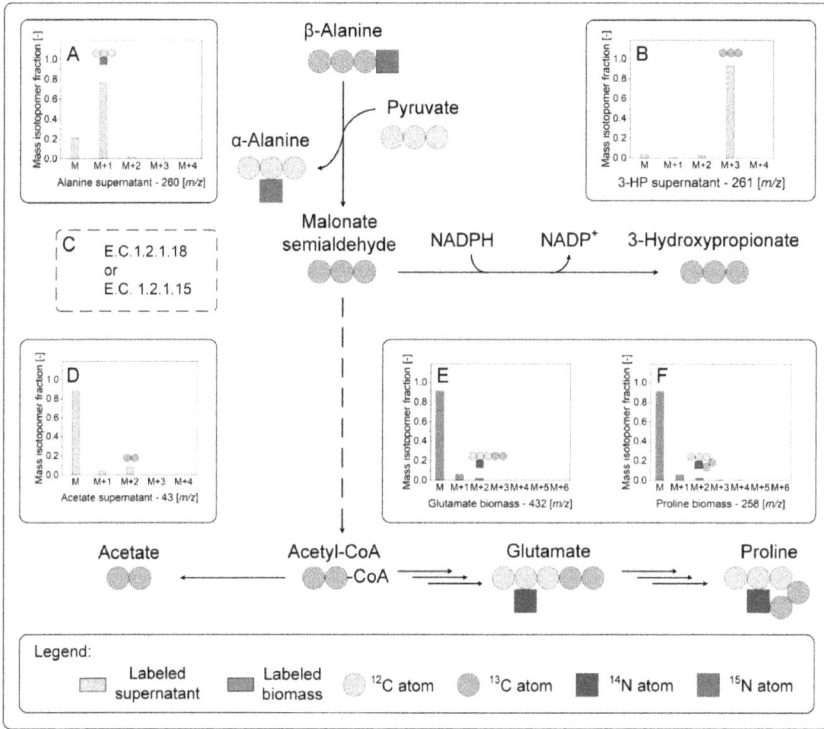

Figure 4.34. Assumed pathway topology of the engineered 3-HP metabolism unraveled by GC-MS. The strain *B. succiniciproducens* DD3 $P_{EM7}panD_{cgl}$-$RBS_{EM7}bapta_{ppu}^+$-$RBS_{EM7}ydfG_{eco}^+$ was cultivated in minimal medium supplemented with ^{13}C-^{15}N-β-alanine. Subsequent GC-MS measurements revealed, that Bapta$_{ppu}$ protein catalyzes the transamination of β-alanine to alanine by use of pyruvate. This was shown by a mass shift in the m+1 mass isotope distribution of alanine (**A**), indicating a labelled amino group transfer. Additionally it can be directly proven that 3-HP originates from the fed β-alanine (**B**). The surplus of consumed β-alanine might relate to the activity of a malonate semialdehyde dehydrogenase, which converts malonate semialdehyde to acetyl-CoA (**C**). The latter was proven by m+2 labelling patterns in acetate (**D**), glutamate (**E**) and proline (**F**), respectively.

95

4.5.6 The codon-optimized $panD_{cgl}^+$ gene enables *De-novo* 3-HP synthesis from glucose

Nonetheless of remaining bottlenecks in the 3-HP synthesis using *B. succiniciproducens*, a third generation producer was designed. The codon-optimization of $panD_{cgl}$ improved β-alanine formation substantially, which could furthermore increase the 3-HP production. Therefore, the 3-HP operon was modified, using $panD_{cgl}^+$, yielding Bsuc_PL98. Subsequent strain construction resulted in *B. succiniciproducens* DD3 + Bsuc_PL98.

The resulting strain was grown in glucose minimal medium under CO_2 atmosphere (**Figure 4.35**). The cells grew from early on, consumed glucose, and showed, as observed before, a constant performance regarding the succinate production (**Figure 4.35 A**).

Cells formed *De-novo* 3-HP from glucose (**Figure 4.35 B**) up to 86 ± 15 mg L^{-1} within 40 h, without supplementation of aspartate or β-alanine. Additionally, only low β-alanine levels indicated an almost complete conversion of this produced precursor (**Figure 4.35 B**). Furthermore, a reduction of the 3-HP titer was observed, when growth ceased. This indicated a back flux into malonate semialdehyde, which is converted as mentioned before.

Taken together, *De-novo* synthesis of 3-HP from glucose was achieved successfully. Further strain engineering appears important for improving 3-HP production. Relevant targets include the deletion of pathways, responsible for the observed carbon loss on the level of malonate semialdehyde. Another drawback is the loss of carbon in the deamination step from β-alanine to malonate semialdehyde, while alanine is formed from pyruvate. Without recovery of the formed alanine, suboptimal yields are unavoidable. Furthermore, improvement in β-alanine synthesis and reduction of succinate production may enhance the 3-HP formation. Therefore, increasing enzymatic activity of PanD, or use of the newly identified PanP protein should be focused on, beside the improvement of aspartate supply. The latter can be achieved by overexpression of the *aspA* gene, as shown recently (Song et al., 2016).

In addition, elimination of succinate formation in *B. succiniciproducens* appears challenging. A *B. succiniciproducens* DD3 *ΔfrdA* derivate strain, lacking fumarate reductase, which transfers electrons to fumarate leading to succinate formation, is unable to grow anaerobically (**Figure 6.12**). When equipped with the 3-HP operon, it was not possible to restore anaerobic growth, although the last step of the pathway comprises a reductive electron transfer step (**Figure 6.13**). This indicates that succinate production of *B. succiniciproducens* is essential for viability under anaerobic conditions, due to redox balancing. Moreover, literature suggests an elementary role of succinate in H^+ efflux in regard of transport issues and energy generation (Choi et al., 2013).

In respect of the investigated literature, this example is a unique demonstration of 3-HP production from glucose in the family of *Pasteurellaceae*.

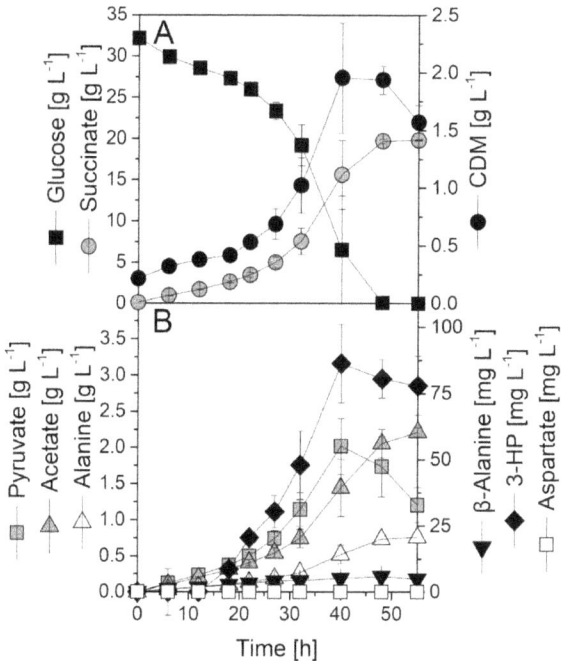

Figure 4.35. Anaerobic growth physiology of a third generation 3-HP producer strain of *B. succiniciproducens* DD3. The strain *B. succiniciproducens* DD3 P_{EM7}-$panD_{cgl}^+$-RBS_{EM7}-$bapta_{ppu}^+$-RBS_{EM7}-$ydfG_{eco}^+$ contains all 3-HP production genes under $EM7^*$ promoter control. Cultivation in glucose minimal medium under CO_2 atmosphere was conducted. The major performance parameters of the strain, i.e. succinate production, were not affected (**A**). A low, but significant, production of 3-HP was observed (**B**). In 40h, up to 86 mg L^{-1} 3-HP was formed. Measurement of organic acids, sugars and amino acids was conducted using HPLC. The data represent three independent replicates with means and standard deviations. CDM, Cell dry mass.

5 CONCLUSION AND OUTLOOK

Without doubt, metabolic engineering of tailor-made producers of industrial relevant chemicals, offers a huge potential to shape a bio-based economy. This is relevant due to the challenges mankind is facing nowadays, i.e. climate change and decreasing supplies of fossil resources. This brings biotechnology in focus of the chemical industry, relying on future strategies for the production of bio-based products and daily goods from renewable feed stocks (Bozell and Petersen, 2010).

B. succiniciproducens, got into the focus of research when the run for commercialization of bio-based succinate, a C_4 organic diacid, was initiated (Becker et al., 2013; Choi et al., 2013; Lange et al., 2017; Werpy et al., 2004). By harnessing the distinct metabolism of *B. succiniciproducens*, providing incorporation of CO_2 while forming succinate, a commercialized process was established by the BASF SE and Corbion Purac. Beside the industrial relevant C_4 acid succinate, C_3 products became relevant, namely 3-hydroxypropionate (Werpy et al., 2004). Less was known about the production capabilities of *Pasteurellaceae*, and in particular *B. succiniciproducens*, regarding C_3 products, which is the focus of this work.

By establishing an advanced genetic engineering tool, by using blue-white screening for genome based engineering of *B. succiniciproducens*, a basis for straightforward strain engineering efforts was laid. It was furthermore demonstrated, that strain selection is possible, using kanamycin. This is essential for more sophisticated genome engineering tools like the recently evoked CRISPR/Cas9 system, using two plasmid systems (Chung et al., 2017). Furthermore, promoter studies enhanced the genetic toolbox for *B. succiniciproducens*, identifying homologous and heterologous candidates for rational gene expression. The latter broadened the toolbox for *B. succiniciproducens* for future metabolic engineering studies using this microbe.

Rational engineering of *B. succiniciproducens* for the production of the C_3 amino acid alanine was conducted as an example project. A strain, containing the deletion of the *ldhA* and *pflD* gene which expresses the alanine dehydrogenase AlaD from *G. stearothermophilus* XL65-6, was assessed for alanine production. This strain formed 0.7 g L^{-1} alanine under aerobic conditions. Alanine production was improved drastically to 29 g L^{-1} in a fed-batch by metabolic and process engineering efforts. Here, xylose was shown to be a superior feedstock, which is advantageous due to its origin from lignocellulosic biomass. Significant performance improvements were generated by the

98

use of anaerobic gas atmospheres, comprising N_2. Application of the latter reduced formation of the main by-products acetate and succinate, enabling an almost exclusive production of alanine by engineered *B. succiniciproducens* ALA-1. These results demonstrate a valuable and unique product shift in the *Pasteurellaceae* family, known for prominent succinate producers, e.g. *A. succinogenes* and *M. succiniciproducens*. More sophisticated engineering strategies, regarding the decrease of specific productivity during the process, can yield a superior alanine producer, being highly competitive to established producers like *E. coli* (Zhou et al., 2015), *C. glutamicum* (Yamamoto et al., 2012) and, recently evoked, *V. natriegens* (Hoffart et al., 2017). A key to success is the understanding of breeding *B. succiniciproducens* to high cell densities, harnessing the outstanding specific glucose uptake rate.

Further genetic engineering was conducted for the recombinant production of an alanine isomer, β-alanine. A combinatorial approach, validating suitable enzymes, i.e. aspartate 1-decarboxylase (PanD) from *E. coli* and *C. glutamicum*, and promoters and their combination was targeted. The latter enabled the *De-novo* β-alanine production of up to 100 mg L^{-1} from glucose, a unique example in the *Pasteurellaceae* family. Here, a heterologous promoter derivative of the commonly known *EM7* promoter was shown to be superior compared to the homologous *pflD* promoter. Furthermore, codon optimization of the *panD_cgl* gene from *C. glutamicum* was the key to success. Additionally, a candidate of the PanP protein family from *V. natriegens* was evaluated as aspartate 1-decarboxylase enzyme and shown to be superior compared to the PanD_cgl enzyme. It was demonstrated, that the specific enzymatic activity of the PanD enzyme was rather low, explaining the low production efficiency in contrast to PanP. Understanding of activity issues, in regard of the cleavage of the PanD protein to its mature and active form in *B. succiniciproducens*, should improve β-alanine production, certainly. Even the identification of stronger promoters, compared to the evaluated set, can improve this issue.

The produced β-alanine was targeted for conversion to 3-HP using engineered *B. succiniciproducens* with the implemented β-alanine route (Valdehuesa et al., 2013). A completely codon-optimized operon, comprising *panD_cgl+*, *bapta_ppu+* and *ydfG_eco+* under *EM7** promoter control, enabled the *De-novo* synthesis of about 100 mg L^{-1} 3-HP under anaerobic conditions. This depicts another unique example, demonstrating the production of C_3 chemicals in the *Pasteurellaceae* family, in particular *B. succiniciproducens*.

The downstream 3-HP production enzymes Bapta$_{ppu}$ and YdfG$_{eco}$, were shown to be sufficiently active in *B. succiniciproducens*. It was demonstrated, that the insufficient PanD enzyme activity hampers 3-HP production, and surplus, the insufficient aspartate supply, as demonstrated during the PanD and PanP enzyme assays. Furthermore, a conversion of malonate semialdehyde into the acetyl-CoA pool was unraveled by use of GC/MS. This is according to the finding, that β-alanine and 3-HP are not metabolized by *B. succiniciproducens*. Only activation of the 3-HP synthesis pathway enabled the drain of β-alanine carbon. It seems challenging to identify the corresponding pathway and responsible enzymes of this drain. But computational analysis suggests, that *putA* (*DD1522*), encoding a putative aldehyde dehydrogenase, is most likely a candidate for such a conversion. Thus it is concluded, that a deletion of the *putA* (*DD1522*) gene is promising to overcome this drain. As mentioned before, without doubt, improving β-alanine production performance will enhance consequently the 3-HP production.

Anaerobic production of β-alanine and 3-HP using *B. succiniciproducens* is accompanied by its natural strong production of succinate. This demonstrates, that lot of carbon is still available for re-routing into the products of interest. However, eliminating succinate production is concluded to be highly challenging. On the one hand, it was shown in this study, that a derivative strain of *B. succiniciproducens* DD3, lacking fumarate reductase (Δ*frdA*), is not able to grow anaerobically. This suggests a somehow distinct and essential role of fumarate reductase for anaerobic growth, transferring electrons on fumarate yielding succinate. It seems likely, that fumarate respiration evolved (Hong et al., 2004) consequently for the CO_2 enriched atmosphere (65 % v/v) of the bovine rumen (Guettler et al., 1999). This is furthermore emphasized by the demonstration, that the implementation of the tested 3-HP synthesis pathway is not able to restore anaerobic growth of this strain. Although the last step, reduction of malonate semialdehyde to 3-HP, comprises an electron transfer. Additionally, the distinct role of succinate in H^+ transport issues, for energy generation, seem to impair the elimination of this prominent product generally (Choi et al., 2013).

As shown, the proof-of-concept of producing C_3 products with *B. succiniciproducens* was successful. Future engineering using the established tools of this work might improve the production performance, to broaden the application field of *B. succiniproducens*.

6 APPENDIX

Table 6.1. Overview of the stock solutions for the preparation of media for cultivation of *B. succiniciproducens*. The specific mixing of the stocks for the different media is given below. All compounds were dissolved in demineralized water to the final volume, and subsequently sterilized as indicated by filtration (s) (Filtropur S 0.2 syringe filter, Sarstedt, Nümbrecht, Germany) or autoclaving (a) for 20 minutes at 121 °C. Vitamin stock 1 solution was prepared by resuspending riboflavin, nicotinic acid and biotin individually in demineralized water followed by dissolving with 6 M NaOH (about 100 µL). Additionally, the remaining vitamins were dissolved and pooled and the pH of the solution was adjusted to pH 7.5. For trace elements, 5 M HCl (Young Lee, 1996) was used as solvent instead of demineralized water. Chloramphenicol for strain selection was dissolved in pure ethanol. The 5-Brom-4-chlor-3-indoxyl-β-D-galactopyranosid (X-gal) stock solution was prepared with dimethylformamid as the solvent.

Stock solution	Compound	Amount [g]	Volume [mL]	Sterilization method
Glucose, 50 %	Glucose·H_2O	25	50	s
Xylose, 50 %	Xylose	25	50	s
Sucrose, 50 %	Sucrose	25	50	s
Fructose, 50 %	Fructose	25	50	s
Glycerol, 50 %	Glycerol	25	50	s
Yeast extract[a], 10 %	Yeast extract	25	250	a
BHI[a], 10 %	BHI	25	250	a
Bacto peptone[a], 10 %	Bacto peptone	25	250	a
Ammonium sulphate, 50 %, pH 7.2[b]	$(NH_4)_2SO_4$	25	50	s
Ammonium sulphate, 50 %	$(NH_4)_2SO_4$	25	50	s
ACES[c], 500 mM, pH 7.2[d]	ACES	91.1	1000	a
Sodium carbonate, 25 %	Na_2CO_3	12.5	50	s
Phosphate, 50 %	K_2HPO_4	25	50	a
Glycine-betaine, 500 mM	Glycine-betaine	2.93	50	s
L-Aspartate, 25 %	L-Aspartate	12.5	50	s
β-Alanine, 25 %	β-Alanine	12.5	50	s
3-HP, 25 %	3-Hydroxypropionate	2.5	10	s
Salt solution, 14 %	NaCl	5		
	$MgCl_2·6H_2O$	1	50	s
	$CaCl_2·6H_2O$	1		
		[mg]	[mL]	
Vitamin stock 1, 100x, pH 7.5[b]	Thiamine·HCl	75		
	Riboflavine	15		
	Nicotinic acid	75		
	Calcium pantothenate	250	25	s
	Pyridoxal·HCl	25		
	Biotin	12.5		
	Cyanocobalamine	1.25		
Trace elements, 200x[e]	$Fe(II)SO_4·7H_2O$	500		
	$Ca(II)Cl_2·2H_2O$	100		
	$Mn(II)SO_4·H_2O$	18.6		
	$Zn(II)SO_4·7H_2O$	110	50	a
	$Cu(II)SO_4·5H_2O$	50		
	$Na_2B_4O_7·10H_2O$	1		
	$(NH_4)_6Mo_7O_{24}·4H_2O$	5		
Chloramphenicol, 5 %[f]	Chloramphenicol	2500	50	s
X-Gal, 8 %[g]	5-Brom-4-chlor-3-indoxyl-β-D-galactopyranosid	400	5	-[h]

[a] Becton and Dickinson
[b] pH adjusted with 1 M NaOH
[c] *N*-(2-Acetamido)-2-aminoethanesulfonic acid
[d] pH adjusted with 6 M NaOH
[e] 5 M HCl as solvent
[f] Ethanol as solvent
[g] Dimethylformamid as solvent
[h] sterilization not necessary

Table 6.2. Codon usage derived from the *B. succiniciproducens* DD1 genome.

Amino acid	Codon	Fraction	Amino acid	Codon	Fraction
Alanine	GCA	0.0862	Leucine	CTA	0.0500
	GCC	0.2342		CTC	0.0400
	GCG	0.2653		CTG	0.1400
	GCT	0.1734		CTT	0.1400
Cysteine	TGC	0.0106		TTA	0.4200
	TGT	0.5105		TTG	0.2100
Aspartate	GAC	0,2984	Lysine	AAA	0,8802
	GAT	0,7016		AAG	0,1198
Arginine	AGA	0.0800	Methionine	ATG	1.0000
	AGG	0.0200	Phenylalanine	TTC	0.3532
	CGA	0.0800		TTT	0.6468
	CGC	0.3000	Proline	CCA	0,0921
	CGG	0.1200		CCC	0,1302
	CGT	0.4000		CCG	0.5200
Asparagine	AAC	0,3691		CCT	0,2580
	AAT	0,6309	Serine	AGC	0.2100
End	TAA	0.0000		AGT	0.1700
	TAG	0.0000		TCA	0,1463
	TGA	0.0000		TCC	0,1952
Glutamine	CAA	0,6591		TCG	0,1399
	CAG	0,3409		TCT	0,1467
Glutamate	GAA	0,8369	Threonine	ACA	0,1722
	GAG	0,1631		ACC	0,3968
Glycine	GGA	0.1300		ACG	0,2221
	GGC	0.3600		ACT	0,2088
	GGG	0.1000	Tryptophan	TGG	1.0000
	GGT	0.4100	Tyrosine	TAC	0,2630
Histidine	CAC	0,3056		TAT	0,7370
	CAT	0,6944	Valine	GTA	0.2700
Isoleucine	ATA	0.0800		GTC	0.1200
	ATC	0.2900		GTG	0.3200
	ATT	0.6300		GTT	0.2900

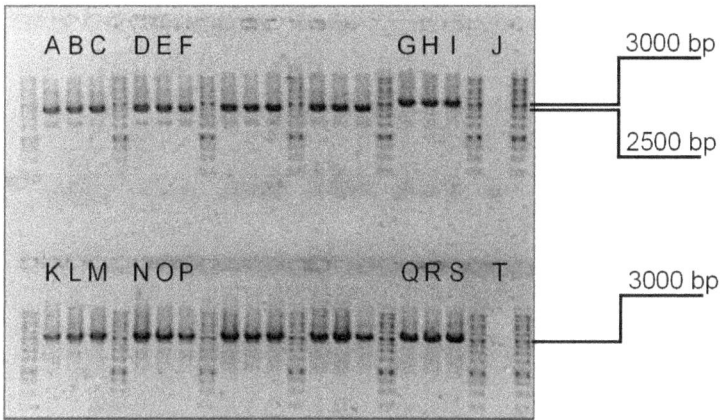

Figure 6.1. Original gel referring to Figure 4.6: Validation of recombinant *B. succiniciproducens* DD3ΔΔ*lacZ* clones. Three individual clones were screened comprising Bsuc_PL94 and Bsuc_PL95 recombinants and the wild type. First recombination in 5' (Lanes A-J) and 3' (Lanes K-T) direction was tested using PCR with the primer pairs P62+63 and P64+65, respectively. Negative controls (Lane J+T) were conducted using demineralized water instead of DNA template. The gel comprised 1 % agarose using a 1 kb DNA ladder for determination of product size.

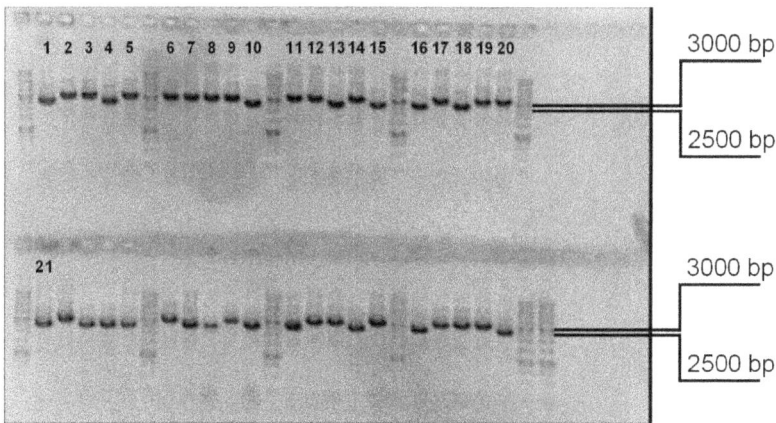

Figure 6.2. Original gel referring to Figure 4.8: Validation of second recombinant clones using blue-white technique and PCR screening. The obtained clones (**A**) were screened by PCR with the 5' integration primer pair P73+74 (**B**). Screening revealed the success of the vector excision from the genome. At least, five out of 18 clones showed the deletion of *DD0789*, namely clone #1, #13, #15, #16 and #18. This is emphasized by comparison to the control clones #4, #10 and #21, which turn blue and contain the plasmid. Detection of amplicons were obtained by agarose gel electrophoresis. The gel comprised 1 % agarose using a 1 kb DNA ladder for determination of product size.

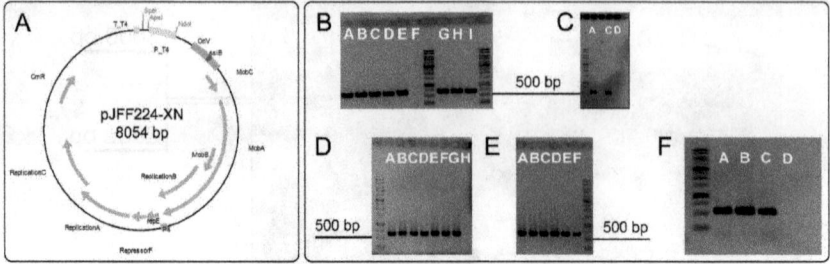

Figure 6.3. Cloning of Bsuc_PL25, Bsuc_PL26 and Bsuc_PL47. All genes were cloned separately under control of the *pflD* or the *EM7** promoter onto linearized (*SpeI* + *ApaI* or *NdeI*) episomal *Pasteurellaceae* vector pJFF224-XN (**A**), yielding Bsuc_PL25, Bsuc_PL26 and Bsuc_PL47, respectively (**B** and **C**). Clones of *Escherichia coli* TOP10 were screened for the correct amplicon of about 650 bp (**B: Lane A-E** - Bsuc_PL25, **Lane G-I** - Bsuc_PL26, **C: Lane A** and **C – Bsuc_PL47**). Transformation of the latter into *Basfia succiniciproducens* DD3 was furthermore successful (**D: Lane A-G** - Bsuc_PL25, **E: Lane A-F** – Bsuc_PL26, **F: Lane A-C** – Bsuc_PL47). Negative controls (**B: Lane F, C: Lane D, F: Lane D**) were conducted using demineralized water instead of DNA template. The gels comprised 1 % agarose using a 1 kb DNA ladder for determination of product size.

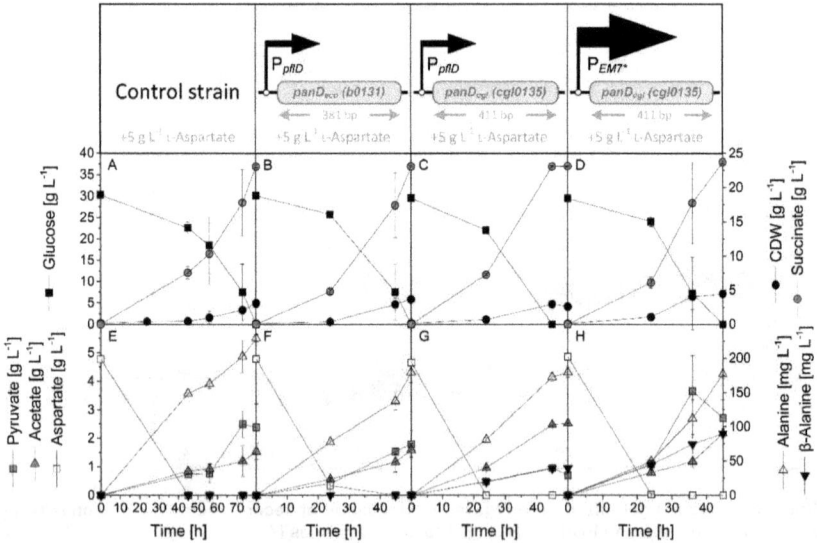

Figure 6.4. Cultivation profiles referring to Figure 4.24. CDW, Cell dry weight.

Sequence 6.1. Sequence of the codon-optimized *panD*_{cgl}⁺ gene from *C. glutamicum* for optimized expression in *B. succiniciproducens*. The gene was synthesized by Thermo Fisher Scientific (Regensburg, Germany)

5'-

ATGTTACGCACCATTTTGGGCAGCAAAATTCATCGTGCGACCGTGACGCAAGCGGATTTAGATTATGTGGGTA
GCGTGACCATTGATGCCGATTTAGTGCATGCGGCAGGTTTAATTGAAGGTGAAAAAGTGGCGATTGTGGATAT
TACCAATGGTGCGCGTTTAGAAACCTATGTGATTGTGGGTGATGCAGGCACCGGTAATATTTGTATTAATGGT
GCGGCAGCGCATTTGATTAATCCGGGTGATTTAGTGATCATCATGAGCTATTTACAAGCGACCGATGCGGAAG
CGAAAGCGTATGAACCGAAAATTGTGCATGTGGATGCGGATAATCGTATTGTGGCGTTAGGTAATGATTTAGC
GGAAGCGTTACCTGGTAGCGGTTTATTAACCAGCCGTAGCATTTAA-3'

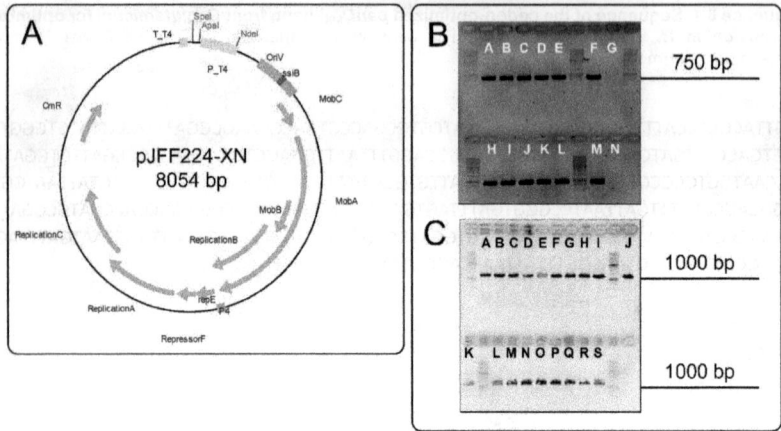

Figure 6.5. Cloning of Bsuc_PL80 and Bsuc_PL86. The codon-optimized *panD$_{cgl}$* gene was cloned under control of P*$_{pflD}$* or P*$_{EM7}$* onto linearized (*NdeI*) episomal *Pasteurellaceae* vector pJFF224-XN (**A**), yielding Bsuc_PL80 and Bsuc_PL86 (**B**). Different pJFF224-XN screening primer pairs were used, yielding differing amplicons. Clones of *Escherichia coli* TOP10 were screened for the correct amplicon of about 750 bp (**B: Lane A-E** - Bsuc_PL80, **Lane H-L** - Bsuc_PL86). Transformation of the latter into *Basfia succiniciproducens* DD3 was furthermore successful as proven by the amplicon at about 1000 bp (**C: Lane A-I** - Bsuc_PL80, **Lane K-R** - Bsuc_PL26). Positive controls (**B:** Lane **F + M**, C: Lane **J + S**) were conducted using Bsuc_PL80 and Bsuc_PL86 as template, respectively. Negative controls (**B: Lane G + N**, **N: Lane D, F: Lane D**) were conducted using demineralized water instead of DNA template. The gels comprised 1 % agarose using a 1 kb DNA ladder for determination of product size.

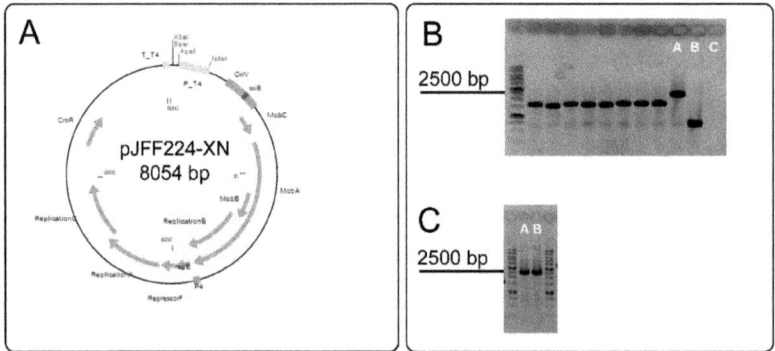

Figure 6.6. Cloning of Bsuc_PL105. The *panP$_{vna}$* gene was cloned under control of P*$_{EM7}$* onto linearized (*XbaI + ApaI*) episomal *Pasteurellaceae* vector pJFF224-XN (**A**), yielding Bsuc_PL105 (**B**). Clones of *Escherichia coli* TOP10 were screened for the correct amplicon of about 2400 bp (**B: Lane A** - Bsuc_PL105, **Lane B** depicts a clone with the empty vector pJFF224-XN). Transformation of the latter into *Basfia succiniciproducens* DD3 was furthermore successful as proven by the amplicon at about 2400 bp (**B: Lane A** - Bsuc_PL105). But only one clone was obtained. Positive control (**C:** Lane **B**) was conducted using Bsuc_PL105 template. Negative control (**B: Lane C**) was conducted using demineralized water instead of DNA template. The gels comprised 1 % agarose using a 1 kb DNA ladder for determination of product size.

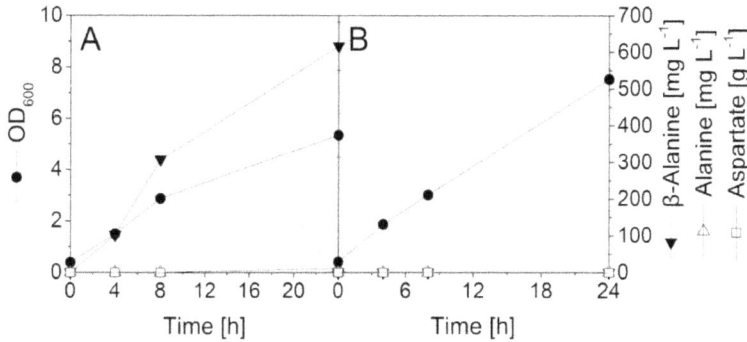

Figure 6.7. Cultivation of *E. coli* DH10B + Bsuc_PL105 in M9 minimal medium expressing a new identified aspartate 1-decarboxylase (PanP$_{vna}$) from *Vibrio natriegens*. The producing strain formed up to 600 mg L^{-1} of β-alanine in 24 h, whereas the control strain, containing the empty vector pJFF224-XN, did not. Measurement of amino acids was conducted using HPLC. The data represent three independent replicates with means and standard deviations.

Table 6.3. Determination of the protein concentration from Pan assay crude extracts. The individual extract was measured three times using the BCA-Assay. Dilutions were made on scale. Protein concentration is given in mg mL^{-1} with mean and standard deviations.

Extract	Protein [mg mL^{-1}] diluted	Dilution Factor	Protein Ø [mg mL^{-1}]	Protein deviation [mg mL^{-1}]
PanD assay				
pJFF224 I	0.765	10.41		
pJFF224 II	0.772	10.12	8.060	0.305
pJFF224 III	0.817	10.28		
Bsuc_PL47 I	0.684	10.43		
Bsuc_PL47 II	0.687	10.16	7.058	0.076
Bsuc_PL47 III	0.683	10.34		
Bsuc_PL80 I	0.734	10.17		
Bsuc_PL80 II	0.718	10.26	7.418	0.051
Bsuc_PL80 III	0.706	10.51		
Bsuc_PL105 I	0.683	10.39		
Bsuc_PL105 II	0.684	10.10	6.986	0.095
Bsuc_PL105 III	0.695	10.01		
PanP assay				
pJFF224 I	0.813	10.90		
pJFF224 II	0.832	10.28	8.658	0.170
pJFF224 III	0.841	10.18		
Bsuc_PL80 I	0.806	10.36		
Bsuc_PL80 II	0.755	10.28	8.051	0.291
Bsuc_PL80 III	0.800	10.05		
Bsuc_PL105 I	0.891	10.25		
Bsuc_PL105 II	0.846	10.29	8.962	0.222
Bsuc_PL105 III	0.890	10.16		
Bsuc_PL105 I	0.813	10.90		
Bsuc_PL105 II	0.832	10.28	8.928[a]	0.255
Bsuc_PL105 III	0.841	10.18		

[a] Crude extract used for PanP assay in **Figure 4.29 E**

107

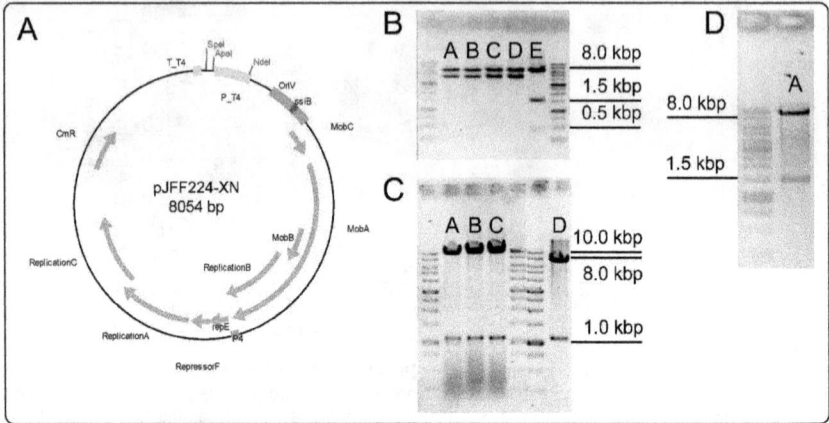

Figure 6.8. Cloning of Bsuc_PL27, Bsuc_PL52 and Bsuc_PL98. *P. putida* KT2440 and *E. coli* K12 MG1655 were chosen as sources for the genes *bapta$_{ppu}$*$^+$ and *ydfG$_{eco}$*$^+$, respectively. Different constructs for heterologous gene expression allowing 3-HP production from glucose were cloned into pJFF224-XN (**A**). Validation of cloning was conducted using restriction enzymes. Validation of Bsuc_PL27 (**B**). Here, the DNA was cut with the enzymes *Sma*I and *Nde*I. The cut site of *Sma*I is located on pJFF224-XN in the chloramphenicol resistance gene and in the multiple cloning site. *Nde*I cuts 358 bp downstream of *Apa*I. Therefore, predicted digestion patterns for Bsuc_PL27 should show a two band pattern (4358 bp and 6164 bp), because the *Sma*I cut site in the multiple cloning site was eliminated due to cloning. The latter was confirmed in the digestion assay (**Lane A-D**). The negative control conducted with pJFF224-XN should yield a three band pattern (410 bp, 1478 bp and 6164 bp), which was observed as well (**Lane E**). Validation of Bsuc_PL52 (**C**). The plasmid Bsuc_PL52 was confirmed by digestion, using *Sph*I. The cut site of *Sph*I is once located in the multiple cloning site of pJFF224-XN 594 bp upstream of *Spe*I. When the *panD$_{cgl}$* gene is fused with the P$_{EM7*}$, a new *Sph*I cut sites arises. Therefore the predicted two band pattern (1105 bp and 9582 bp) for Bsuc_P52 was observed (**Lane A-C**). The plasmid Bsuc_PL47 (P*EM7*panD$_{cgl}$*) was used as negative control (1105 bp and 7452 bp) (**Lane D**). Validation of Bsuc_PL98 (**D**). The construct Bsuc_PL98 was confirmed in a more convenient way. Here, *Mun*I was used, which cuts in *bapta$_{ppu}$* and furthermore in the *ydfG$_{eco}$* gene. The predicted two band pattern (1500 bp and 9187 bp), was observed and confirmed the cloning success (**Lane A**). All plasmids were constructed successfully. The gels comprised 1 % agarose using a 1 kb DNA ladder for determination of product size.

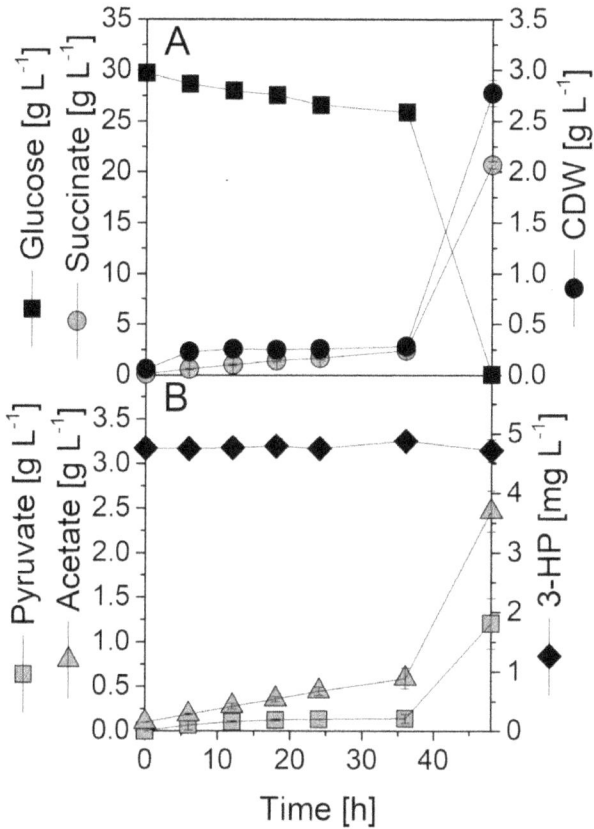

Figure 6.9. Cultivation profiles referring to Figure 4.31. CDW, Cell dry weight.

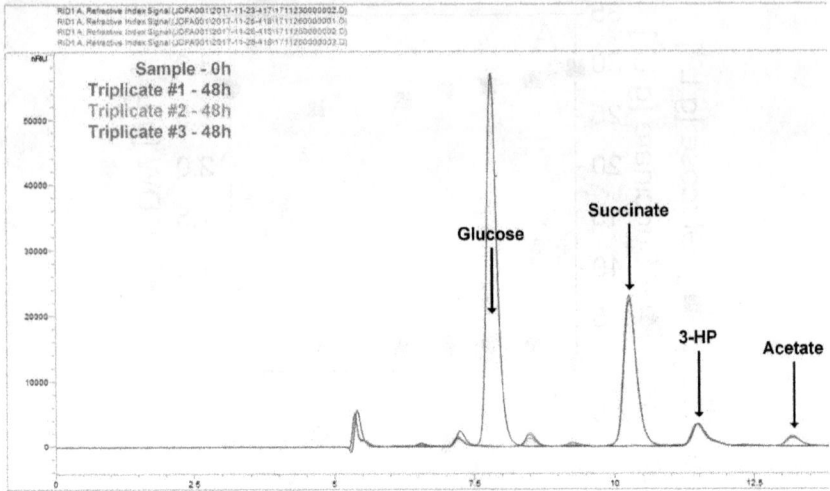

Figure 6.10. 3-HP conversion test. *B. succiniciproducens* DD3 + pJFF224-XN was grown in presence of 5 g L^{-1} 3-HP. Overlay of the 0h and 48 h sample showed clearly, that 3-hydroxypropionate is not converted by *B. succiniciproducens*.

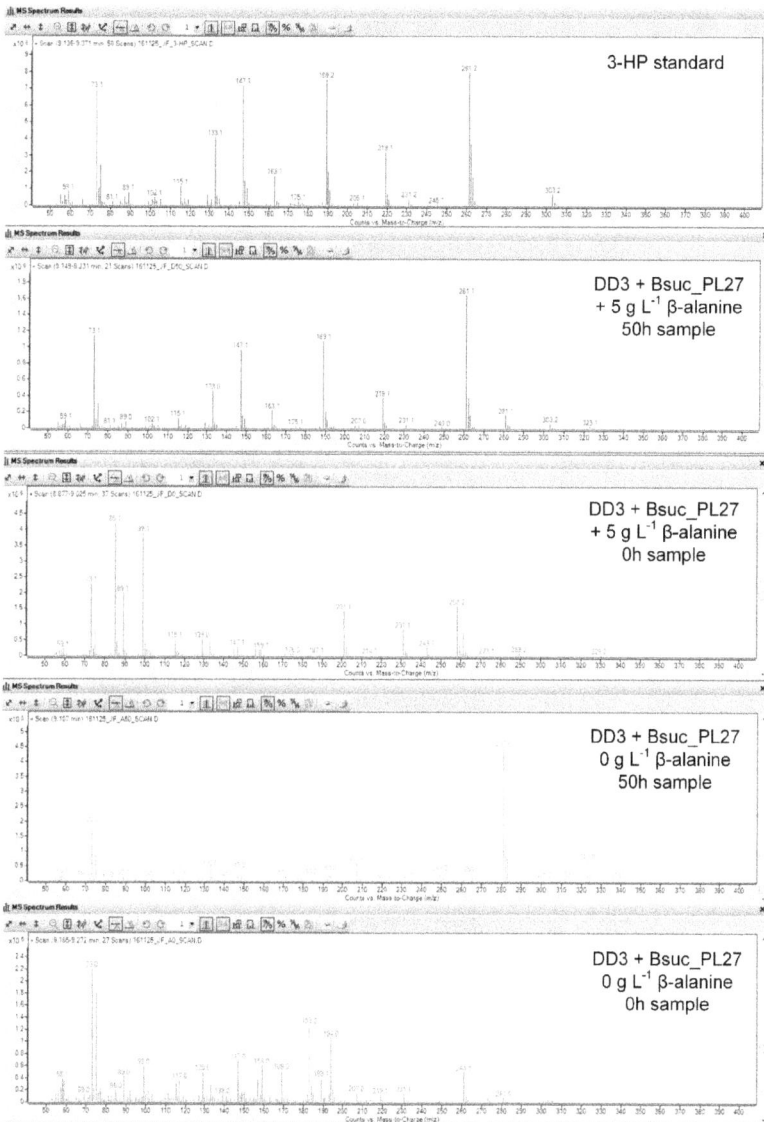

Figure 6.11. GC-MS measurements of *B. succiniciproducens* cultivation supernatants. The samples were measured in scan mode (50 – 400 *m/z*). Measurement of the 3-HP standard contained the main 3-HP ions at 73 *m/Z*, 133 *m/z*, 147 *m/z*, 189 *m/z*, 219 *m/z*, 261 *m/z* and 303 *m/z* covered by the 3-HP peak (retention time: 9.2 min). Presence of the 3-HP ions was shown in the 3-HP producing strain *B. succiniciproducens* DD3 + Bsuc_PL27 in the 50 h sample which converted the β-alanine. In contrast, when β-alanine was not supplied, the 50 h sample did not show any signs of 3-HP in the supernatant.

111

Table 6.4. Mass isotopomer distribution (MID) for tracer experiments using $^{13}C^{15}N$-β-alanine. Samples of naturally labeled ($^{12}C^{14}N$-β-alanine) supernatant (A50) and biomass (A50) and labeled ($^{13}C^{15}N$-β-alanine) supernatant (B50) and biomass (B50) were taken after 50h, when glucose was completely consumed during cultivation. A naturally labeled standard containing the examined compounds was additionally measured. Where indicated, data is not available (-).

Analyte	m/z	Mass isotopomer	Standard sample (S)	Unlabeled supernatant A50	Unlabeled biomass A50	Labeled supernatant B50	Labeled biomass B50
Lactate	261.2	M	0.75	-	0.74	-	0.74
		M+1	0.17	-	0.17	-	0.17
		M+2	0.07	-	0.07	-	0.07
		M+3	0.01	-	0.01	-	0.01
3-HP	261.2	M	0.75	0.75	0.74	0.04	0.15
		M+1	0.17	0.17	0.17	0.01	0.05
		M+2	0.07	0.07	0.08	0.03	0.04
		M+3	0.01	0.01	0.02	0.92	0.76
Succinate	289.2	M	0.74	0.74	0.74	0.73	0.73
		M+1	0.17	0.18	0.18	0.18	0.18
		M+2	0.07	0.07	0.07	0.07	0.07
		M+3	0.01	0.01	0.01	0.01	0.01
		M+4	0.00	0.00	0.00	0.00	0.00
β-Alanine	260.2	M	0.75	0.75	0.74	0.00	0.02
		M+1	0.17	0.17	0.17	0.00	0.01
		M+2	0.07	0.07	0.07	0.11	0.15
		M+3	0.01	0.01	0.01	0.05	0.06
		M+4	0.00	0.00	0.00	0.83	0.75
Alanine	260.2	M	0.74	0.74	0.74	0.17	0.35
		M+1	0.17	0.17	0.17	0.62	0.48
		M+2	0.07	0.07	0.07	0.15	0.12
		M+3	0.01	0.01	0.01	0.06	0.04
		M+4	0.00	0.00	0.00	0.01	0.01
Glycine	246.2	M	0.76	-	0.75	-	0.74
		M+1	0.16	-	0.17	-	0.17
		M+2	0.07	-	0.07	-	0.07
		M+3	0.01	-	0.01	-	0.01
Valine	288.2	M	0.73	-	0.73	-	0.72
		M+1	0.19	-	0.18	-	0.19
		M+2	0.07	-	0.07	-	0.07
		M+3	0.01	-	0.01	-	0.01
		M+4	0.00	-	0.00	-	0.00
		M+5	0.00	-	0.00	-	0.00
		M+6	0.00	-	0.00	-	0.00
Leucine	302.3	M	0.72	-	0.72	-	0.69
		M+1	0.19	-	0.19	-	0.19
		M+2	0.07	-	0.07	-	0.09
		M+3	0.01	-	0.01	-	0.02
		M+4	0.00	-	0.00	-	0.00
		M+5	0.00	-	0.00	-	0.00
		M+6	0.00	-	0.00	-	0.00
		M+7	0.00	-	0.00	-	0.00
Isoleucine	302.3	M	0.72	-	0.72	-	0.71
		M+1	0.19	-	0.19	-	0.20
		M+2	0.07	-	0.07	-	0.08
		M+3	0.01	-	0.01	-	0.01
		M+4	0.00	-	0.00	-	0.00
		M+5	0.00	-	0.00	-	0.00
		M+6	0.00	-	0.00	-	0.00
		M+7	0.00	-	0.00	-	0.00
Proline	258.2	M	0.73	-	0.73	-	0.70
		M+1	0.18	-	0.18	-	0.18
		M+2	0.07	-	0.07	-	0.09
		M+3	0.01	-	0.01	-	0.02
		M+4	0.00	-	0.00	-	0.00
		M+5	0.00	-	0.00	-	0.00
Serine	390.3	M	0.64	-	0.64	-	0.64
		M+1	0.22	-	0.22	-	0.23
		M+2	0.10	-	0.10	-	0.10
		M+3	0.02	-	0.02	-	0.02
		M+4	0.01	-	0.01	-	0.01

Table 6.4. MID for tracer experiments using $^{13}C^{15}N$-β-alanine. Continued 1.

Analyte	m/z	Mass isotopomer	Standard sample (S)	Unlabeled supernatant A50	Unlabeled biomass A50	Labeled supernatant B50	Labeled biomass B50
Threonine	404.4	M	0.64	-	0.64	-	0.63
		M+1	0.23	-	0.23	-	0.23
		M+2	0.10	-	0.10	-	0.11
		M+3	0.02	-	0.02	-	0.03
		M+4	0.01	-	0.01	-	0.01
		M+5	0.00	-	0.00	-	0.00
Phenyl-alanine	336.3	M	0.70	-	0.70	-	0.68
		M+1	0.21	-	0.20	-	0.21
		M+2	0.08	-	0.08	-	0.08
		M+3	0.01	-	0.01	-	0.02
		M+4	0.00	-	0.00	-	0.00
		M+5	0.00	-	0.00	-	0.00
		M+6	0.00	-	0.00	-	0.00
		M+7	0.00	-	0.00	-	0.00
		M+8	0.00	-	0.00	-	0.00
		M+9	0.00	-	0.00	-	0.00
		M+10	0.00	-	0.00	-	0.00
Aspartate	418.4	M	0.64	-	0.63	-	0.63
		M+1	0.23	-	0.23	-	0.23
		M+2	0.11	-	0.11	-	0.11
		M+3	0.02	-	0.03	-	0.03
		M+4	0.01	-	0.01	-	0.01
		M+5	0.00	-	0.00	-	0.00
Glutamate	432.4	M	0.63	-	0.63	-	0.60
		M+1	0.23	-	0.23	-	0.23
		M+2	0.11	-	0.11	-	0.12
		M+3	0.03	-	0.03	-	0.03
		M+4	0.01	-	0.01	-	0.01
		M+5	0.00	-	0.00	-	0.00
		M+6	0.00	-	0.00	-	0.00
Lysine	431.4	M	0.62	-	0.61	-	0.59
		M+1	0.24	-	0.23	-	0.24
		M+2	0.11	-	0.11	-	0.12
		M+3	0.03	-	0.03	-	0.03
		M+4	0.01	-	0.01	-	0.01
		M+5	0.00	-	0.00	-	0.00
		M+6	0.00	-	0.00	-	0.00
		M+7	0.00	-	0.00	-	0.00
		M+8	0.00	-	0.00	-	0.00
Tyrosine	466.4	M	0.60	-	0.60	-	0.59
		M+1	0.25	-	0.25	-	0.25
		M+2	0.11	-	0.11	-	0.11
		M+3	0.03	-	0.03	-	0.03
		M+4	0.01	-	0.01	-	0.01
		M+5	0.00	-	0.00	-	0.00
		M+6	0.00	-	0.00	-	0.00
		M+7	0.00	-	0.00	-	0.00
		M+8	0.00	-	0.00	-	0.00
		M+9	0.00	-	0.00	-	0.00
		M+10	0.00	-	0.00	-	0.00
Acetate	43.1	M	0.92	0.92	-	0.87	-
		M+1	0.03	0.03	-	0.03	-
		M+2	0.02	0.02	-	0.08	-

Table 6.5. Mass isotopomer distribution (MID) for tracer experiments using $^{13}C^{15}N$-β-alanine corrected for natural labeling. Samples of naturally labeled ($^{12}C^{14}N$-β-alanine) supernatant (A50) and biomass (A50) and labeled ($^{13}C^{15}N$-β-alanine) supernatant (B50) and biomass (B50) were taken after 50h, when glucose was completely consumed during cultivation. A naturally labeled standard containing the examined compounds was additionally measured. Where indicated, data is not available (-).

Analyte	m/z	Mass isotopomer	Standard sample (S)	Unlabeled supernatant A50	Unlabeled biomass A50	Labeled supernatant B50	Labeled biomass B50
Lactate	261.2	M	0.97	-	0.96	-	0.96
		M+1	0.03	-	0.03	-	0.04
		M+2	0.00	-	0.00	-	0.00
		M+3	0.00	-	0.00	-	0.00
3-HP	261.2	M	0.97	0.97	0.95	0.04	0.16
		M+1	0.03	0.03	0.03	0.01	0.02
		M+2	0.00	0.00	0.01	0.03	0.03
		M+3	0.00	0.00	0.00	0.93	0.79
Succinate	289.2	M	0.96	0.95	0.95	0.95	0.95
		M+1	0.04	0.04	0.04	0.05	0.05
		M+2	0.00	0.00	0.00	0.00	0.00
		M+3	0.00	0.00	0.00	0.00	0.00
		M+4	0.00	0.00	0.00	0.00	0.00
β-Alanine	260.2	M	0.97	0.97	0.96	0.18	0.18
		M+1	0.03	0.03	0.03	0.13	0.12
		M+2	0.00	0.00	0.00	0.32	0.36
		M+3	0.00	0.00	0.00	0.38	0.34
		M+4	-	-	-	-	-
Alanine	260.2	M	0.96	0.96	0.96	0.21	0.46
		M+1	0.03	0.03	0.04	0.76	0.53
		M+2	0.00	0.00	0.00	0.02	0.02
		M+3	0.00	0.00	0.00	0.00	0.00
		M+4	0.00	0.00	0.00	0.00	0.00
Glycine	246.2	M	0.98	-	0.97	-	0.96
		M+1	0.02	-	0.03	-	0.04
		M+2	0.00	-	0.00	-	0.00
		M+3	0.00	-	0.00	-	0.00
Valine	288.2	M	0.94	-	0.95	-	0.93
		M+1	0.06	-	0.05	-	0.06
		M+2	0.00	-	0.00	-	0.00
		M+3	0.00	-	0.00	-	0.00
		M+4	0.00	-	0.00	-	0.00
		M+5	0.00	-	0.00	-	0.00
		M+6	0.00	-	0.00	-	0.00
Leucine	302.3	M	0.97	-	0.97	-	0.94
		M+1	0.03	-	0.03	-	0.04
		M+2	0.00	-	0.00	-	0.02
		M+3	0.00	-	0.00	-	0.00
		M+4	0.00	-	0.00	-	0.00
		M+5	0.00	-	0.00	-	0.00
		M+6	0.00	-	0.00	-	0.00
		M+7	0.00	-	0.00	-	0.00
Isoleucine	302.3	M	0.97	-	0.97	-	0.96
		M+1	0.03	-	0.02	-	0.03
		M+2	0.00	-	0.00	-	0.00
		M+3	0.00	-	0.00	-	0.00
		M+4	0.00	-	0.00	-	0.00
		M+5	0.00	-	0.00	-	0.00
		M+6	0.00	-	0.00	-	0.00
		M+7	0.00	-	0.00	-	0.00
Proline	258.2	M	0.95	-	0.95	-	0.91
		M+1	0.05	-	0.05	-	0.06
		M+2	0.00	-	0.00	-	0.03
		M+3	0.00	-	0.00	-	0.00
		M+4	0.00	-	0.00	-	0.00
		M+5	-	-	-	-	-
Serine	390.3	M	0.97	-	0.97	-	0.96
		M+1	0.03	-	0.03	-	0.04
		M+2	0.00	-	0.00	-	0.00
		M+3	0.00	-	0.00	-	0.00
		M+4	0.00	-	0.00	-	0.00

Table 6.5. Mass isotopomer distribution (MID) for tracer experiments using $^{13}C^{15}N$-β-alanine corrected for natural labeling. Continued 1.

Analyte	m/z	Mass isotopomer	Standard sample (S)	Unlabeled supernatant A50	Unlabeled biomass A50	Labeled supernatant B50	Labeled biomass B50
Threonine	404.4	M	0.96	-	0.96	-	0.95
		M+1	0.04	-	0.04	-	0.05
		M+2	0.00	-	0.00	-	0.00
		M+3	0.00	-	0.00	-	0.00
		M+4	0.00	-	0.00	-	0.00
		M+5	0.00	-	0.00	-	0.00
Phenyl-alanine	336.3	M	0.91	-	0.91	-	0.89
		M+1	0.09	-	0.08	-	0.10
		M+2	0.00	-	0.00	-	0.01
		M+3	0.00	-	0.00	-	0.00
		M+4	0.00	-	0.00	-	0.00
		M+5	0.00	-	0.00	-	0.00
		M+6	0.00	-	0.00	-	0.00
		M+7	0.00	-	0.00	-	0.00
		M+8	0.00	-	0.00	-	0.00
		M+9	0.00	-	0.00	-	0.00
		M+10	0.00	-	0.00	-	0.00
Aspartate	418.4	M	0.96	-	0.96	-	0.95
		M+1	0.04	-	0.04	-	0.05
		M+2	0.00	-	0.00	-	0.00
		M+3	0.00	-	0.00	-	0.00
		M+4	0.00	-	0.00	-	0.00
		M+5	0.00	-	0.00	-	0.00
Glutamate	432.4	M	0.95	-	0.95	-	0.91
		M+1	0.05	-	0.05	-	0.06
		M+2	0.00	-	0.00	-	0.02
		M+3	0.00	-	0.00	-	0.00
		M+4	0.00	-	0.00	-	0.00
		M+5	0.00	-	0.00	-	0.00
		M+6	0.00	-	0.00	-	0.00
Lysine	431.4	M	0.94	-	0.92	-	0.89
		M+1	0.06	-	0.06	-	0.08
		M+2	0.00	-	0.01	-	0.02
		M+3	0.00	-	0.00	-	0.00
		M+4	0.00	-	0.00	-	0.00
		M+5	0.00	-	0.00	-	0.00
		M+6	0.00	-	0.00	-	0.00
		M+7	0.00	-	0.00	-	0.00
		M+8	-	-	-	-	-
Tyrosine	466.4	M	0.78	-	0.90	-	0.89
		M+1	0.07	-	0.09	-	0.10
		M+2	0.00	-	0.01	-	0.01
		M+3	0.00	-	0.00	-	0.00
		M+4	0.00	-	0.00	-	0.00
		M+5	0.00	-	0.00	-	0.00
		M+6	0.04	-	0.00	-	0.00
		M+7	0.04	-	0.00	-	0.00
		M+8	0.04	-	0.00	-	0.00
		M+9	0.04	-	0.00	-	0.00
		M+10	0.00	-	0.00	-	0.00
Acetate	43.1	M	0.92	0.92	-	0.87	-
		M+1	0.03	0.03	-	0.03	-
		M+2	0.02	0.02	-	0.08	-

115

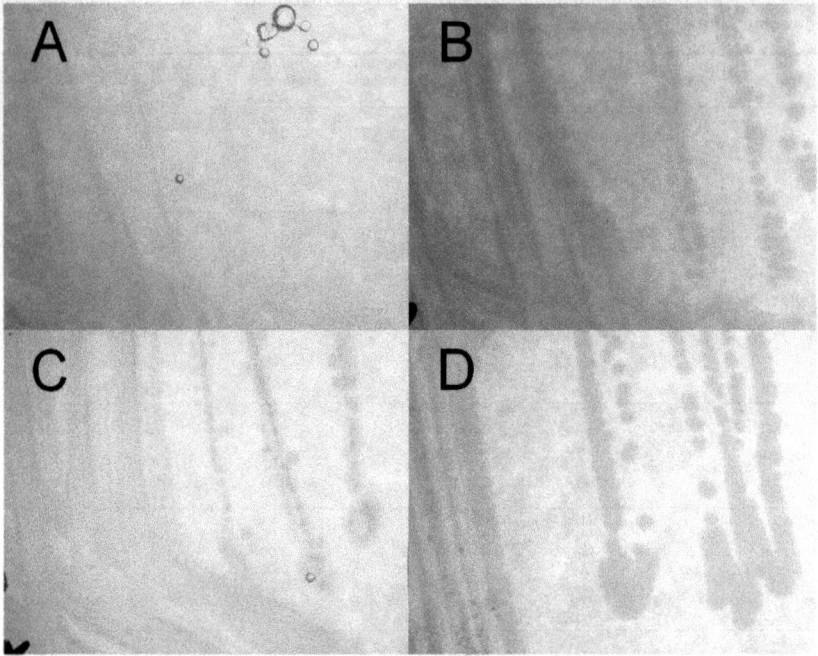

Figure 6.12. Comparison of aerobic and anaerobic growth of *B. succiniciproducens* strains. The strains were streaked on buffered BHI agarplates. Incubation was conducted at 37 °C for 48 h. The strain *B. succiniciproducens* DD3 pH 5.3 Δ*frdA* showed impaired growth under anaerobic conditions (**A**). In contrast, normal growth was observed under aerobic conditions (**B**). The parent strain *B. succiniciproducens* DD3 pH 5.3, lacking the *ldhA* and the *pflD* gene showed normal growth, either under anaerobic (**C**) or aerobic conditions (**D**).

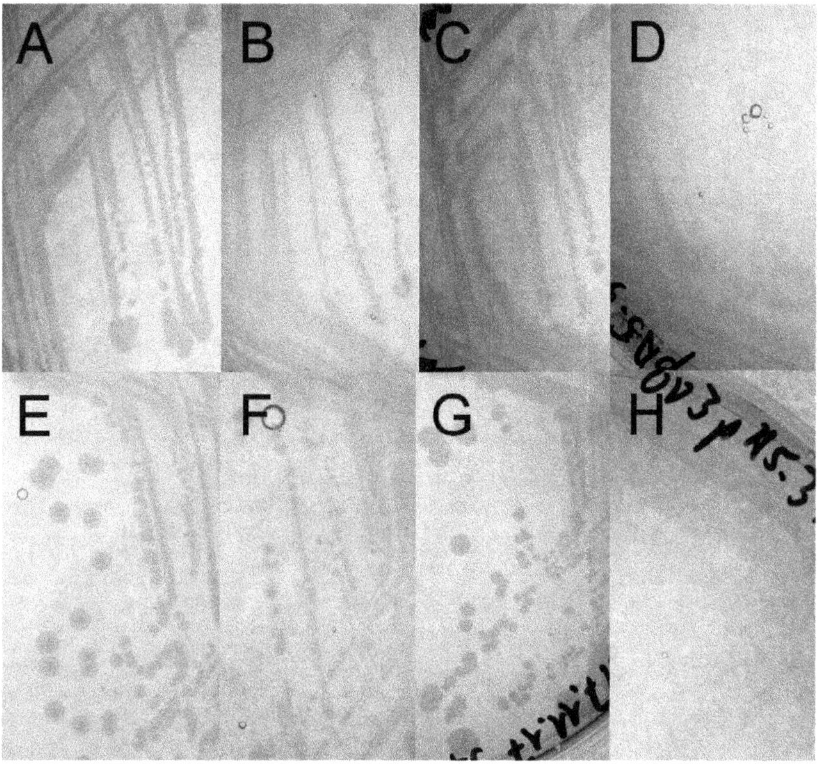

Figure 6.13. Comparison of *B. succiniciproducens* **DD3 and DD3 pH5.3Δ*ldhA*::*aspA* Δ*frdA*::*asd* containing the plasmids pJFF224 and Bsuc_PL98 under aerobic and anaerobic growth conditions.** Cells were streaked on buffered BHI agar plates, which were incubated up to 72h under aerobic, or anaerobic conditions. The DD3 strain showed growth. DD3 + pJFF224 aerob (**A**) and anaerob (**B**). DD3 + Bsuc_PL98 aerob (**E**) and anaerob (**F**). DD3 pH5.3Δ*ldhA*::*aspA* Δ*frdA*::*asd* + pJFF224 aerob (**C**) and anaerob (**D**). DD3 pH5.3Δ*ldhA*::*aspA* Δ*frdA*::*asd* + Bsuc_PL98 aerob (**G**) and anaerob (**H**).

6.1 Figure index

6.2 Table index

7 BIBLIOGRAPHY

Adler, P., Bolten, C.J., Dohnt, K., Hansen, C.E., Wittmann, C., (2013) Core Fluxome and Metafluxome of Lactic Acid Bacteria under Simulated Cocoa Pulp Fermentation Conditions. Applied and Environmental Microbiology 79, 5670-5681.

Aimi, J., Badylak, J., Williams, J., Chen, Z.D., Zalkin, H., Dixon, J.E., (1990) Cloning of a cDNA encoding adenylosuccinate lyase by functional complementation in Escherichia coli. Journal of Biological Chemistry 265, 9011-9014.

Alonso, S., Rendueles, M., Díaz, M., (2014) Microbial production of specialty organic acids from renewable and waste materials. Critical Reviews in Biotechnology, 1-17.

Alper, H., Fischer, C., Nevoigt, E., Stephanopoulos, G., (2005) Tuning genetic control through promoter engineering. PNAS 102, 12678-12683.

Andersen, K.B., von Meyenburg, K., (1980) Are growth rates of Escherichia coli in batch cultures limited by respiration? Journal of Bacteriology 144, 114-123.

Barton, N., (2015) Molekularbiologische Studien mit Basfia succiniciproducens zur Optimierung der Stammentwicklung. Institute of Systems Biotechnology. Saarland University, Saarbrücken.

Beauprez, J.J., De Mey, M., Soetaert, W.K., (2010) Microbial succinic acid production: Natural versus metabolic engineered producers. Process Biochemistry 45, 1103-1114.

Becker, J., Klopprogge, C., Herold, A., Zelder, O., Bolten, C.J., Wittmann, C., (2007) Metabolic flux engineering of L-lysine production in Corynebacterium glutamicum - over expression and modification of G6P dehydrogenase. J. Biotechnol. 132, 99-109.

Becker, J., Lange, A., Fabarius, J., Wittmann, C., (2015) Top value platform chemicals: bio-based production of organic acids. Curr. Opin. Biotechnol. 36, 168-175.

Becker, J., Reinefeld, J., Stellmacher, R., Schäfer, R., Lange, A., Meyer, H., Lalk, M., Zelder, O., von Abendroth, G., Schröder, H., Häfner, S., Wittmann, C., (2013) Systems-wide analysis and engineering of metabolic pathway fluxes in bio-succinate producing Basfia succiniciproducens. Biotechnol. Bioeng. 110, 3013-3023.

Becker, J., Wittmann, C., (2012a) Bio-based production of chemicals, materials and fuels – Corynebacterium glutamicum as versatile cell factory. Current Opinion in Biotechnology 23, 631-640.

Becker, J., Wittmann, C., (2012b) Systems and synthetic metabolic engineering for amino acid production – the heartbeat of industrial strain development. Curr. Opin. Biotechnol. 23, 718-726.

Becker, J., Wittmann, C., (2015) Advanced Biotechnology: Metabolically Engineered Cells for the Bio-Based Production of Chemicals and Fuels, Materials, and Health-Care Products. Angewandte Chemie International Edition 54, 3328-3350.

Becker, J., Zelder, O., Häfner, S., Schröder, H., Wittmann, C., (2011) From zero to hero - Design-based systems metabolic engineering of Corynebacterium glutamicum for L-lysine production. Metab. Eng. 13, 159-168.

Borodina, I., Kildegaard, K.R., Jensen, N.B., Blicher, T.H., Maury, J., Sherstyk, S., Schneider, K., Lamosa, P., Herrgard, M.J., Rosenstand, I., Oberg, F., Forster, J., Nielsen, J., (2015) Establishing a synthetic pathway for high-level production of 3-hydroxypropionic acid in Saccharomyces cerevisiae via beta-alanine. Metab. Eng. 27, 57-64.

Bozell, J.J., Petersen, G.R., (2010) Technology development for the production of biobased products from biorefinery carbohydrates-the US Department of Energy's "Top 10" revisited. Green Chemistry 12, 539-554.

Buschke, N., Schafer, R., Becker, J., Wittmann, C., (2013) Metabolic engineering of industrial platform microorganisms for biorefinery applications--optimization of substrate spectrum and process robustness by rational and evolutive strategies. Bioresource Technology 135, 544-554.

Chen, C., Ding, S., Wang, D., Li, Z., Ye, Q., (2014) Simultaneous saccharification and fermentation of cassava to succinic acid by *Escherichia coli* NZN111. Bioresource Technology 163, 100-105.

Cheng, K.K., Wang, G.Y., Zeng, J., Zhang, J.A., (2013) Improved succinate production by metabolic engineering. BioMed research international 2013, 538790.

Choi, S., Kim, H.U., Kim, T.Y., Kim, W.J., Lee, M.H., Lee, S.Y., (2013) Production of 4-hydroxybutyric acid by metabolically engineered *Mannheimia succiniciproducens* and its conversion to gamma-butyrolactone by acid treatment. Metab. Eng. 20, 73-83.

Choi, S., Song, C.W., Shin, J.H., Lee, S.Y., (2015) Biorefineries for the production of top building block chemicals and their derivatives. Metab. Eng. 28, 223-239.

Choi, S., Song, H., Lim, S.W., Kim, T.Y., Ahn, J.H., Lee, J.W., Lee, M.-H., Lee, S.Y., (2016) Highly selective production of succinic acid by metabolically engineered *Mannheimia succiniciproducens* and its efficient purification. Biotechnol. Bioeng. 113, 2168-2177.

Chu, H.S., Kim, Y.S., Lee, C.M., Lee, J.H., Jung, W.S., Ahn, J.-H., Song, S.H., Choi, I.S., Cho, K.M., (2015) Metabolic engineering of 3-hydroxypropionic acid biosynthesis in *Escherichia coli*. Biotechnol. and Bioeng. 112, 356-364.

Chung, M.-E., Yeh, I.H., Sung, L.-Y., Wu, M.-Y., Chao, Y.-P., Ng, I.S., Hu, Y.-C., (2017) Enhanced integration of large DNA into *E. coli* chromosome by CRISPR/Cas9. Biotechnol. Bioeng. 114, 172-183.

Cimini, D., Argenzio, O., D'Ambrosio, S., Lama, L., Finore, I., Finamore, R., Pepe, O., Faraco, V., Schiraldi, C., (2016) Production of succinic acid from *Basfia succiniciproducens* up to the pilot scale from *Arundo donax* hydrolysate. Bioresource Technology 222, 355-360.

Cormack, B.P., Valdivia, R.H., Falkow, S., (1996) FACS-optimized mutants of the green fluorescent protein (GFP). Gene 173, 33-38.

Crutzen, P.J., (2002) The "anthropocene". J. Phys. IV France 12, 1-5.

De Mey, M., Maertens, J., Lequeux, G.J., Soetaert, W.K., Vandamme, E.J., (2007) Construction and model-based analysis of a promoter library for *E. coli*: an indispensable tool for metabolic engineering. BMC Biotech. 7, 1-14.

Dlugokencky, E., Tans, P., (2017) (online reference) Trends in atmospheric carbon dioxide. NOAA's Earth System Research Laboratory. https://www.esrl.noaa.gov/gmd/ccgg/trends/global.html.

Dousse, F., Thomann, A., Brodard, I., Korczak, B.M., Schlatter, Y., Kuhnert, P., Miserez, R., Frey, J., (2008) Routine Phenotypic Identification of Bacterial Species of the Family *Pasteurellaceae* Isolated from Animals. Journal of Veterinary Diagnostic Investigation 20, 716-724.

Drocourt, D., Reynes, J.P., Tiraby, G., (2007) Synthetic genes and bacterial plasmids devoid of CpG. Google Patents.

Dusch, N., Pühler, A., Kalinowski, J., (1999) Expression of the *Corynebacterium glutamicum panD* Gene Encoding L-Aspartate-α-Decarboxylase Leads to Pantothenate Overproduction in *Escherichia coli*. Applied and Environmental Microbiology 65, 1530-1539.

Fabarius, J., (2013) Entwicklung alaninproduzierender Stämme von *Basfia succiniciproducens* für Fermentationsprozesse mit Hilfe des Metabolic Engineering., Institute of Biochemical Engineering. University of Stuttgart, Stuttgart.

Fernández-Llamosas, H., Castro, L., Blázquez, M.L., Díaz, E., Carmona, M., (2017) Speeding up bioproduction of selenium nanoparticles by using *Vibrio natriegens* as microbial factory. Sci. Rep. 7, 16046.

Fernie, A.R., Carrari, F., Sweetlove, L.J., (2004) Respiratory metabolism: glycolysis, the TCA cycle and mitochondrial electron transport. Current Opinion in Plant Biology 7, 254-261.

Fotheringham, I.G., Dacey, S.A., Taylor, P.P., Smith, T.J., Hunter, M.G., Finlay, M.E., Primrose, S.B., Parker, D.M., Edwards, R.M., (1986) The cloning and sequence analysis of the *aspC* and *tyrB* genes from *Escherichia coli* K12. Comparison of the primary structures of the aspartate aminotransferase and aromatic aminotransferase of *E. coli* with those of the pig aspartate aminotransferase isoenzymes. Biochemical Journal 234, 593-604.

Frey, J., (1992) Construction of a broad host range shuttle vector for gene cloning and expression in *Actinobacillus pleuropneumoniae* and other *Pasteurellaceae*. Res. Microbiol. 143, 263-269.

Fujisawa, H., Nagata, S., Misono, H., (2003) Characterization of short-chain dehydrogenase/reductase homologues of *Escherichia coli* (*YdfG*) and *Saccharomyces cerevisiae* (*YMR226C*). Biochimica et Biophysica Acta (BBA) - Proteins and Proteomics 1645, 89-94.

Geng, S., Tian, Q., An, S., Pan, Z., Chen, X., Jiao, X., (2016) High-Efficiency, Two-Step Scarless–Markerless Genome Genetic Modification in *Salmonella enterica*. Curr. Microbiol. 72, 700-706.

Germano, G.J., Anderson, K.E., (1968) Purification and properties of L-alanine dehydrogenase from *Desulfovibrio desulfuricans*. J. Bacteriol. 96, 55-60.

Gibson, D.G., Young, L., Chuang, R.-Y., Venter, J.C., Hutchison, C.A., Smith, H.O., (2009) Enzymatic assembly of DNA molecules up to several hundred kilobases. Nat. Methods 6, 343-345.

Grabar, T.B., Zhou, S., Shanmugam, K.T., Yomano, L.P., Ingram, L.O., (2006) Methylglyoxal bypass identified as source of chiral contamination in L(+) and D(−)-lactate fermentations by recombinant *Escherichia coli*. Biotechnol. Lett. 28, 1527-1535.

Guettler, M.V., Jain, M.K., Rumler, D., (1996) Method for making succinic acid, bacterial variants for use in the process, and methods for obtaining variants. In: Institute, M.B. (Ed.).

Guettler, M.V., Rumler, D., Jain, M.K., (1999) *Actinobacillus succinogenes sp. nov.*, a novel succinic-acid-producing strain from the bovine rumen. Int. J. Syst. Bacteriol. 1, 207-216.

Hayaishi, O., Nishizuka, Y., Tatibana, M., Takeshita, M., Kuno, S., (1961) Enzymatic Studies on the Metabolism of β-Alanine. Journal of Biological Chemistry 236, 781-790.

Hoffart, E., Grenz, S., Lange, J., Nitschel, R., Müller, F., Schwentner, A., Feith, A., Lenfers-Lücker, M., Takors, R., Blombach, B., (2017) High substrate uptake rates empower *Vibrio natriegens* as production host for industrial biotechnology. Appl. Environ. Microbiol.

Hong, S.H., Kim, J.S., Lee, S.Y., In, Y.H., Choi, S.S., Rih, J.K., Kim, C.H., Jeong, H., Hur, C.G., Kim, J.J., (2004) The genome sequence of the capnophilic rumen bacterium *Mannheimia succiniciproducens*. Nat. Biotechnol. 22, 1275-1281.

Huang, Y., Li, Z., Shimizu, K., Ye, Q., (2013) Co-production of 3-hydroxypropionic acid and 1,3-propanediol by *Klebseilla pneumoniae* expressing *aldH* under microaerobic conditions. Bioresource Technology 128, 505-512.

Ingram, C.U., Bommer, M., Smith, M.E.B., Dalby, P.A., Ward, J.M., Hailes, H.C., Lye, G.J., (2007) One-pot synthesis of amino-alcohols using a de-novo transketolase and β-alanine: Pyruvate transaminase pathway in *Escherichia coli*. Biotechnol. Bioeng. 96, 559-569.

Inoue, H., Nojima, H., Okayama, H., (1990) High efficiency transformation of *Escherichia coli* with plasmids. Gene 96, 23-28.

Jang, Y.S., Jung, Y.R., Lee, S.Y., Kim, J.M., Lee, J.W., Oh, D.B., Kang, H.A., Kwon, O., Jang, S.H., Song, H., Lee, S.J., Kang, K.Y., (2007) Construction and characterization of shuttle vectors for succinic acid-producing rumen bacteria. Appl. Environ. Microbiol. 73, 5411-5420.

Jansen, M.L., van Gulik, W.M., (2014) Towards large scale fermentative production of succinic acid. Curr. Opin. Biotechnol. 30, 190-197.

Jiang, M., Wan, Q., Liu, R., Liang, L., Chen, X., Wu, M., Zhang, H., Chen, K., Ma, J., Wei, P., Ouyang, P., (2014) Succinic acid production from corn stalk hydrolysate in an *E. coli* mutant generated by atmospheric and room-temperature plasmas and metabolic evolution strategies. Journal of Industrial Microbiology & Biotechnology 41, 115-123.

Jojima, T., Fujii, M., Mori, E., Inui, M., Yukawa, H., (2010) Engineering of sugar metabolism of *Corynebacterium glutamicum* for production of amino acid L-alanine under oxygen deprivation. Applied Microbiology and Biotechnology 87, 159-165.

Joshi, R.V., Schindler, B.D., McPherson, N.R., Tiwari, K., Vieille, C., (2014) Development of a Markerless Knockout Method for *Actinobacillus succinogenes*. Applied and Environmental Microbiology 80, 3053-3061.

Keasling, J.D., (2010) Manufacturing molecules through metabolic engineering. Science 330, 1355-1358.

Kiernan, J.A., (2007) Indigogenic substrates for detection and localization of enzymes. Biotechnic & Histochemistry 82, 73-103.

Kim, D.Y., Yim, S.C., Lee, P.C., Lee, W.G., Lee, S.Y., Chang, H.N., (2004) Batch and continuous fermentation of succinic acid from wood hydrolysate by *Mannheimia succiniciproducens* MBEL55E. Enzyme. Microb. Tech. 35, 648-653.

Kim, K., Kim, S.K., Park, Y.C., Seo, J.H., (2014) Enhanced production of 3-hydroxypropionic acid from glycerol by modulation of glycerol metabolism in recombinant *Escherichia coli*. Bioresource Technology 156, 170-175.

Kim, T.Y., Kim, H.U., Song, H., Lee, S.Y., (2009) In silico analysis of the effects of H_2 and CO_2 on the metabolism of a capnophilic bacterium *Mannheimia succiniciproducens*. J. Biotechnol. 144, 184-189.

Kim, W.J., Ahn, J.H., Kim, H.U., Kim, T.Y., Lee, S.Y., (2017) Metabolic engineering of *Mannheimia succiniciproducens* for succinic acid production based on elementary mode analysis with clustering. Biotechnology Journal 12.

Konst, P.M., Franssen, M.C.R., Scott, E.L., Sanders, J.P.M., (2009) A study on the applicability of L-aspartate [small alpha]-decarboxylase in the biobased production of nitrogen containing chemicals. Green Chemistry 11, 1646-1652.

Krömer, J.O., Fritz, M., Heinzle, E., Wittmann, C., (2005) In vivo quantification of intracellular amino acids and intermediates of the methionine pathway in *Corynebacterium glutamicum*. Anal. Biochem. 340, 171-173.

Kuhnert, P., Scholten, E., Häfner, S., Mayor, D., Frey, J., (2010) *Basfia succiniciproducens gen. nov., sp. nov.,* a new member of the family *Pasteurellaceae* isolated from bovine rumen. Int. J. Syst. Evol. Microbiol. 60, 44-50.

Kwon, Y.D., Kim, S., Lee, S.Y., Kim, P., (2011) Long-term continuous adaptation of *Escherichia coli* to high succinate stress and transcriptome analysis of the tolerant strain. Journal of bioscience and bioengineering 111, 26-30.

Lange, A., Becker, J., Schulze, D., Cahoreau, E., Portais, J.-C., Haefner, S., Schröder, H., Krawczyk, J., Zelder, O., Wittmann, C., (2017) Bio-based succinate from sucrose: High-resolution 13C metabolic flux analysis and metabolic engineering of the rumen bacterium *Basfia succiniciproducens*. Metab. Eng. 44, 198-212.

Lee, E.-G., Kim, S., Oh, D.-B., Lee, S.Y., Kwon, O., (2012) Distinct Roles of β-Galactosidase Paralogues of the Rumen Bacterium *Mannheimia succiniciproducens*. Journal of Bacteriology 194, 426-436.

Lee, H.H., Ostrov, N., Wong, B.G., Gold, M.A., Khalil, A., Church, G.M., (2016) *Vibrio natriegens*, a new genomic powerhouse. bioRxiv, https://doi.org/10.1101/058487.

Lee, J.W., Choi, S., Kim, J.M., Lee, S.Y., (2010) *Mannheimia succiniciproducens* Phosphotransferase System for Sucrose Utilization. Applied and Environmental Microbiology 76, 1699-1703.

Lee, P.C., Lee, S.Y., Hong, S.H., Chang, H.N., (2002) Isolation and characterization of a new succinic acid-producing bacterium, *Mannheimia succiniciproducens* MBEL55E, from bovine rumen. Appl. Microbiol. Biotechnol. 58, 663-668.

Lee, S.J., Song, H., Lee, S.Y., (2006) Genome-Based Metabolic Engineering of *Mannheimia succiniciproducens* for Succinic Acid Production. Applied and Environmental Microbiology 72, 1939-1948.

Lenz, D., Rothschild, M.A., Kröner, L., (2008) Intoxications due to Ingestion of γ-Butyrolactone: Organ Distribution of γ-Hydroxybutyric Acid and γ-Butyrolactone. Therapeutic Drug Monitoring 30, 755-761.

Leonardi, R., Jackowski, S., (2007) Biosynthesis of Pantothenic Acid and Coenzyme A. EcoSal Plus 2, 4.

Li, C., Tao, F., Ni, J., Wang, Y., Yao, F., Xu, P., (2015) Enhancing the light-driven production of D-lactate by engineering cyanobacterium using a combinational strategy. Sci. Rep. 5.

Li, N., Zhang, B., Chen, T., Wang, Z., Tang, Y.-j., Zhao, X., (2013) Directed pathway evolution of the glyoxylate shunt in *Escherichia coli* for improved aerobic succinate production from glycerol. Journal of Industrial Microbiology & Biotechnology 40, 1461-1475.

Li, Y., Chen, J., Lun, S.-Y., (2001) Biotechnological production of pyruvic acid. Applied Microbiology and Biotechnology 57, 451-459.

Liang, L.-Y., Zheng, Y.-G., Shen, Y.-C., (2008) Optimization of β-alanine production from β-aminopropionitrile by resting cells of *Rhodococcus sp.* G20 in a bubble column reactor using response surface methodology. Process Biochemistry 43, 758-764.

Litsanov, B., Brocker, M., Bott, M., (2012) Toward homosuccinate fermentation: metabolic engineering of *Corynebacterium glutamicum* for anaerobic production of succinate from glucose and formate. Applied and Environmental Microbiology 78, 3325-3337.

Liu, Z.S., Rempel, G.L., (1997) Preparation of superabsorbent polymers by crosslinking acrylic acid and acrylamide copolymers. Journal of Applied Polymer Science 64, 1345-1353.

Long, C.P., Gonzalez, J.E., Cipolla, R.M., Antoniewicz, M.R., (2017) Metabolism of the fast-growing bacterium *Vibrio natriegens* elucidated by 13C metabolic flux analysis. Metab. Eng. 44, 191-197.

Luli, G.W., Strohl, W.R., (1990) Comparison of growth, acetate production, and acetate inhibition of *Escherichia coli* strains in batch and fed-batch fermentations. Applied and Environmental Microbiology 56, 1004-1011.

Lynch, M.D., Gill, R.T., Lipscomb, T.E.W., (2015) Methods for producing 3-hydroxypropionic acid and other products. In: The Regents Of The University Of Colorado, O.B., Inc. (Ed.).

Maida, I., Bosi, E., Perrin, E., Papaleo, M.C., Orlandini, V., Fondi, M., Fani, R., Wiegel, J., Bianconi, G., Canganella, F., (2013) Draft Genome Sequence of the Fast-Growing Bacterium *Vibrio natriegens* Strain DSMZ 759. Genome Announcements 1.

Maleki, N., Eiteman, M., (2017) Recent Progress in the Microbial Production of Pyruvic Acid. Fermentation 3, 8.

McKinlay, J.B., Vieille, C., Zeikus, J.G., (2007) Prospects for a bio-based succinate industry. Applied Microbiology and Biotechnology 76, 727-740.

Mullis, K., Faloona, F., Scharf, S., Saiki, R., Horn, G., Erlich, H., (1986) Specific enzymatic amplification of DNA in vitro: the polymerase chain reaction. Cold Spring Harb. Symp. Quant. Biol. 1, 263-273.

Nassis, G.P., Sporer, B., Stathis, C.G., (2017) β-alanine efficacy for sports performance improvement: from science to practice. British Journal of Sports Medicine 51, 626-627.

Oikawa, T., (2007) Alanine, Aspartate, and Asparagine Metabolism in Microorganisms. In: Wendisch, V.F. (Ed.), Amino Acid Biosynthesis ~ Pathways, Regulation and Metabolic Engineering. Springer Berlin Heidelberg, Berlin, Heidelberg, pp. 273-288.

Okino, S., Noburyu, R., Suda, M., Jojima, T., Inui, M., Yukawa, H., (2008) An efficient succinic acid production process in a metabolically engineered *Corynebacterium glutamicum* strain. Applied Microbiology and Biotechnology 81, 459-464.

Pan, S., Nikolakakis, K., Adamczyk, P.A., Pan, M., Ruby, E.G., Reed, J.L., (2017) Model-enabled gene search (MEGS) allows fast and direct discovery of enzymatic and transport gene functions in the marine bacterium *Vibrio fischeri*. Journal of Biological Chemistry 292, 10250-10261.

Pateraki, C., Patsalou, M., Vlysidis, A., Kopsahelis, N., Webb, C., Koutinas, A.A., Koutinas, M., (2016) *Actinobacillus succinogenes*: Advances on succinic acid production and prospects for development of integrated biorefineries. Biochem. Eng. J. 112, 285-303.

Raspor, P., Goranovič, D., (2008) Biotechnological Applications of Acetic Acid Bacteria. Critical Reviews in Biotechnology 28, 101-124.

Rathnasingh, C., Raj, S.M., Jo, J.E., Park, S., (2009) Development and evaluation of efficient recombinant *Escherichia coli* strains for the production of 3-hydroxypropionic acid from glycerol. Biotechnol. Bioeng. 104, 729-739.

Rogsch, A., (2015) Analysis of potentially constitutive promoters in *Pseudomonas putida* KT2440. Institute of Systems Biotechnology. Saarland University, Saarbrücken.

Rytter, J.V., Helmark, S., Chen, J., Lezyk, M.J., Solem, C., Jensen, P.R., (2014) Synthetic promoter libraries for *Corynebacterium glutamicum*. Appl. Microbiol. Biotechnol. 98, 2617-2623.

Sakanyan, V., Petrosyan, P., Lecocq, M., Boyen, A., Legrain, C., Demarez, M., Hallet, J.-N., Glansdorff, N., (1996) Genes and enzymes of the acetyl cycle of arginine biosynthesis in Corynebacterium glutamicum: enzyme evolution in the early steps of the arginine pathway. Microbiology 142, 99-108.

Salvachúa, D., Smith, H., St. John, P.C., Mohagheghi, A., Peterson, D.J., Black, B.A., Dowe, N., Beckham, G.T., (2016) Succinic acid production from lignocellulosic hydrolysate by *Basfia succiniciproducens*. Bioresource Technology 214, 558-566.

Sambrook, J., and Russell, D. W., (2001) Molecular cloning - A laboratory manual., New York.

Sawers, G., Böck, A., (1988) Anaerobic regulation of pyruvate formate-lyase from *Escherichia coli* K-12. J. Bacteriol. 170, 5330-5336.

Schindler, B.D., Joshi, R.V., Vieille, C., (2014) Respiratory glycerol metabolism of *Actinobacillus succinogenes* 130Z for succinate production. J. Ind. Microbiol. Biotechnol. 41, 1339-1352.

Scholten, E., Dägele, D., (2008) Succinic acid production by a newly isolated bacterium. Biotechnol. Lett. 30, 2143-2146.

Scholten, E., Renz, T., Thomas, J., (2009) Continuous cultivation approach for fermentative succinic acid production from crude glycerol by *Basfia succiniciproducens* DD1. Biotechnol. Lett. 31, 1947-1951.

Schuster, S., Dandekar, T., Fell, D.A., (1999) Detection of elementary flux modes in biochemical networks: a promising tool for pathway analysis and metabolic engineering. Trends in Biotechnology 17, 53-60.

Shen, Y., Zhao, L., Li, Y., Zhang, L., Shi, G., (2014) Synthesis of β-alanine from L-aspartate using L-aspartate-α-decarboxylase from *Corynebacterium glutamicum*. Biotechnology Letters 36, 1681-1686.

Smith, P.K., Krohn, R.I., Hermanson, G.T., Mallia, A.K., Gartner, F.H., Provenzano, M.D., Fujimoto, E.K., Goeke, N.M., Olson, B.J., Klenk, D.C., (1985) Measurement of protein using bicinchoninic acid. Anal. Biochem. 150, 76-85.

Song, C.W., Kim, J.W., Cho, I.J., Lee, S.Y., (2016) Metabolic Engineering of *Escherichia coli* for the Production of 3-Hydroxypropionic Acid and Malonic Acid through beta-Alanine Route. ACS Synthetic Biology.

Song, C.W., Lee, J., Ko, Y.-S., Lee, S.Y., (2015) Metabolic engineering of *Escherichia coli* for the production of 3-aminopropionic acid. Metab. Eng. 30, 121-129.

Speltz, E.B., Regan, L., (2013) White and green screening with circular polymerase extension cloning for easy and reliable cloning. Protein Science : A Publication of the Protein Society 22, 859-864.

Stellmacher, R., Hangebrauk, J., Wittmann, C., Scholten, E., von Abendroth, G., (2010) Fermentative Herstellung von Bernsteinsäure mit *Basfia succiniciproducens* DD1 in Serumflaschen. Chemie Ingenieur Technik 82, 1223-1229.

Stevenson, I.L., (1978) The production of extracellular amino acids by rumen bacteria. Can. J. Microbiol. 24, 1236-1241.

Stuecker, T.N., Tucker, A.C., Escalante-Semerena, J.C., (2012) *PanM*, an acetyl-coenzyme A sensor required for maturation of L-aspartate decarboxylase (*PanD*). MBio 3.

Szenk, M., Dill, K.A., de Graff, A.M.R., (2017) Why Do Fast-Growing Bacteria Enter Overflow Metabolism? Testing the Membrane Real Estate Hypothesis. Cell Systems 5, 95-104.

Takisawa, K., Ooi, T., Matsumoto, K.i., Kadoya, R., Taguchi, S., (2017) Xylose-based hydrolysate from eucalyptus extract as feedstock for poly(lactate-co-3-hydroxybutyrate) production in engineered *Escherichia coli*. Process Biochem. 54, 102-105.

Tsuge, Y., Yamamoto, S., Kato, N., Suda, M., Vertès, A.A., Yukawa, H., Inui, M., (2015) Overexpression of the phosphofructokinase encoding gene is crucial for achieving high production of D-lactate in *Corynebacterium glutamicum* under oxygen deprivation. Appl. Microbiol. Biotechnol. 99, 4679-4689.

UNEP, (2017) The Emissions Gap Report 2017. United Nations Environment Programme (UNEP), Nairobi.

Valdehuesa, K.N., Liu, H., Nisola, G.M., Chung, W.J., Lee, S.H., Park, S.J., (2013) Recent advances in the metabolic engineering of microorganisms for the production of 3-hydroxypropionic acid as C3 platform chemical. Appl. Microbiol. Biotechnol. 97, 3309-3321.

Van Dyk, J.S., Pletschke, B.I., (2012) A review of lignocellulose bioconversion using enzymatic hydrolysis and synergistic cooperation between enzymes—Factors affecting enzymes, conversion and synergy. Biotechnology Advances 30, 1458-1480.

van Maris, A.J.A., Geertman, J.-M.A., Vermeulen, A., Groothuizen, M.K., Winkler, A.A., Piper, M.D.W., van Dijken, J.P., Pronk, J.T., (2004) Directed Evolution of Pyruvate Decarboxylase-Negative *Saccharomyces cerevisiae*, Yielding a C2-Independent, Glucose-Tolerant, and Pyruvate-Hyperproducing Yeast. Applied and Environmental Microbiology 70, 159-166.

van Winden, W.A., Wittmann, C., Heinzle, E., Heijnen, J.J., (2002) Correcting mass isotopomer distributions for naturally occurring isotopes. Biotechnol. Bioeng. 80.

Vemuri, G.N., Eiteman, M.A., Altman, E., (2002) Succinate production in dual-phase *Escherichia coli* fermentations depends on the time of transition from aerobic to anaerobic conditions. Journal of industrial microbiology & biotechnology 28, 325-332.

Vieira, J., Messing, J., (1982) The pUC plasmids, an M13mp7-derived system for insertion mutagenesis and sequencing with synthetic universal primers. Gene 19, 259-268.

Wang, W., Poland, B.W., Honzatko, R.B., Fromm, H.J., (1995) Identification of Arginine Residues in the Putative L-Aspartate Binding Site of Escherichiacoli Adenylosuccinate Synthetase. Journal of Biological Chemistry 270, 13160-13163.

Weinstock, M.T., Hesek, E.D., Wilson, C.M., Gibson, D.G., (2016) Vibrio natriegens as a fast-growing host for molecular biology. Nat. Meth. 13, 849-851.

Werpy T., P.G., Jones S., White J., Aden A., Bozell J., Holladay J., Manheim A., Eliot D., Lasure L., (2004) Top value added chemicals from biomass. Volume I - Results of screening for potential candidates from sugars and synthesis gas. U.S. D. o. Energy, 1-76.

Wieschalka, S., Blombach, B., Bott, M., Eikmanns, B.J., (2013) Bio-based production of organic acids with Corynebacterium glutamicum. Microb. Biotechnol. 6, 87-102.

Wittmann, C., (2007) Fluxome analysis using GC-MS. Microb. Cell Fact. 6, 1-17.

Wittmann, C., Hans, M., Heinzle, E., (2002) In vivo analysis of intracellular amino acid labelings by GC/MS. Anal. Biochem. 307, 379-382.

Xi, Y.-l., Chen, K.-q., Dai, W.-y., Ma, J.-f., Zhang, M., Jiang, M., Wei, P., Ouyang, P.-K., (2013) Succinic acid production by Actinobacillus succinogenes NJ113 using corn steep liquor powder as nitrogen source. Bioresource Technology 136, 775-779.

Xu, K., Xu, P., (2014) Efficient production of L-lactic acid using co-feeding strategy based on cane molasses/glucose carbon sources. Bioresource Technology 153, 23-29.

Yamamoto, S., Gunji, W., Suzuki, H., Toda, H., Suda, M., Jojima, T., Inui, M., Yukawa, H., (2012) Overexpression of genes encoding glycolytic enzymes in Corynebacterium glutamicum enhances glucose metabolism and alanine production under oxygen deprivation conditions. Appl. Environ. Microbiol. 78, 4447-4457.

Yamane, T., Tanaka, R., (2013) Highly accumulative production of L(+)-lactate from glucose by crystallization fermentation with immobilized Rhizopus oryzae. Journal of Bioscience and Bioengineering 115, 90-95.

Yan, D., Wang, C., Zhou, J., Liu, Y., Yang, M., Xing, J., (2014) Construction of reductive pathway in Saccharomyces cerevisiae for effective succinic acid fermentation at low pH value. Bioresource Technology 156, 232-239.

Yang, F., Hanna, M.A., Sun, R., (2012) Value-added uses for crude glycerol--a byproduct of biodiesel production. Biotechnology for Biofuels 5, 13.

Yang, Y.T., Bennett, G.N., San, K.Y., (2001) The effects of feed and intracellular pyruvate levels on the redistribution of metabolic fluxes in Escherichia coli. Metab. Eng. 3, 115-123.

Young Lee, S.Y.L., (1996) Enhanced production of poly(3-hydroxybutyrate) by filamentation-suppressed recombinant Escherichia coli in a defined medium. J. envir. poly. degr. 4, 131-134.

Zahorski, B., (1913) Method of producing citric acid. Google Patents.

Zhang, X., Jantama, K., Moore, J.C., Shanmugam, K.T., Ingram, L.O., (2007) Production of L-alanine by metabolically engineered Escherichia coli. Appl. Microbiol. Biotechnol. 77, 355-366.

Zhou, L., Deng, C., Cui, W.-J., Liu, Z.-M., Zhou, Z.-M., (2015) Efficient L-Alanine production by a thermo-regulated switch in Escherichia coli. Appl. Biochem. Biotechnol., 1-14.

Zhu, X., Tan, Z., Xu, H., Chen, J., Tang, J., Zhang, X., (2014) Metabolic evolution of two reducing equivalent-conserving pathways for high-yield succinate production in *Escherichia coli*. Metab. eng. 24, 87-96.

Zhu, Y., Eiteman, M.A., Altman, R., Altman, E., (2008) High glycolytic flux improves pyruvate production by a metabolically engineered *Escherichia coli* strain. Appl. Environ. Microbiol. 74, 6649-6655.

www.ingramcontent.com/pod-product-compliance
Lightning Source LLC
Chambersburg PA
CBHW060319220326
41598CB00027B/4367